Advancing Your Yoga Practice:

THE ART OF SLOWING DOWN

Advancing Your Yoga Practice:
The Art of Slowing Down

Other books by Susi Hately Aldous:

Anatomy and Asana: Preventing Yoga Injuries
Anatomy and Asana: The Sacroiliac Joints
Anatomy and Asana: The Knees
Anatomy and Asana: The Shoulder Girdle
Yoga for the Desk Jockey™
Therapeutic Yoga for the Shoulders and Hips

Free PDF downloads compiled by Susi Hately Aldous:

One Piece of Advice for Getting Out of Pain, Improving Functional Movement, and Finding Quiet, Ease, and Peace

One Piece of Advice for Being a Great Yoga Teacher

Audio CD by Susi Hately Aldous:

Finding Quiet

Upcoming DVD by Susi Hately Aldous:

Yoga for Cancer Survivors

Other books produced by Functional Synergy:

Yoga for the Core by Suzette O'Byrne

www.functionalsynergy.com

www.anatomyandasana.com

www.yogaforthedeskjockey.com

Advancing Your Yoga Practice:

the Art *of* Slowing Down

FIRST EDITION

Text by Susi Hately Aldous
Photographs by Marnie Burkhart,
Jazhart Studios
Illustrations by Teresa McLaren

Published by Functional Synergy Press

Editors: Andrea Kennedy, Caroline Woods
Book design: Janine Eliana MacKinnon
Printed in Canada by Apache Printing

DISCLAIMER

The purpose of this book is to provide information on the subject of therapeutic yoga. The book does not offer any medical advice to the reader and is not intended as a replacement for appropriate health care and treatment. For such advice, readers should consult their health care practitioners.

Even though this book has 2 authors, many more eyes, ears, bodies and minds helped to bring it to fruition.

From Susi ... Thank you!

To all my students and clients – all of you – you keep teaching me what it means to be a teacher!

Yoga instructors Catherine Townley, Tyla Arnason, and Linda Crawford who practiced the manuscript and provided feedback.

Andrea Kennedy and Caroline Woods for their editing and insights.

Teresa McLaren for beautiful anatomical drawings.

Janine Eliana MacKinnon, who is an amazing graphic designer.

Shala MacKenzie for managing, handling and massaging the office and my day-to-day flow.

Leonor Mowry for following her heart and weaving in the principles of Anatomy and Asana and yoga therapeutics into her practice both as a teacher and student.

Dave, the great guy who is my amazing husband and who inspires me to learn and grow.

Sadie, my furry friend who is always ready for a walk and run.

From Leonor ... Thank you!

To the amazing students who continually inspire me to keep learning and growing.

To the Village Yoga faculty: Jasmin, Annabel, Emma, Marinella, Alex, Lauren and Janice. To work with and be supported by such well-intentioned, talented women is purely and simply, a gift.

To Greg Soucie, my partner in love, life and fun.

To Susi Hately Aldous, friend, teacher and collaborator in "keeping it real"!

And from both of us to you, thank you for picking up this book. We hope it inspires your practice.

Happy exploring,
Susi and Leonor

namaste

I HONOUR THE PLACE IN YOU
WHERE THE ENTIRE UNIVERSE
RESIDES.

I HONOUR THE PLACE IN
YOU OF LIGHT, LOVE, TRUTH,
PEACE, AND WISDOM.

I HONOUR THE PLACE IN
YOU WHERE, WHEN YOU
ARE IN THAT PLACE
AND I AM IN THAT PLACE,
THERE'S ONLY ONE OF US.

—GANDHI

Table *of* Contents

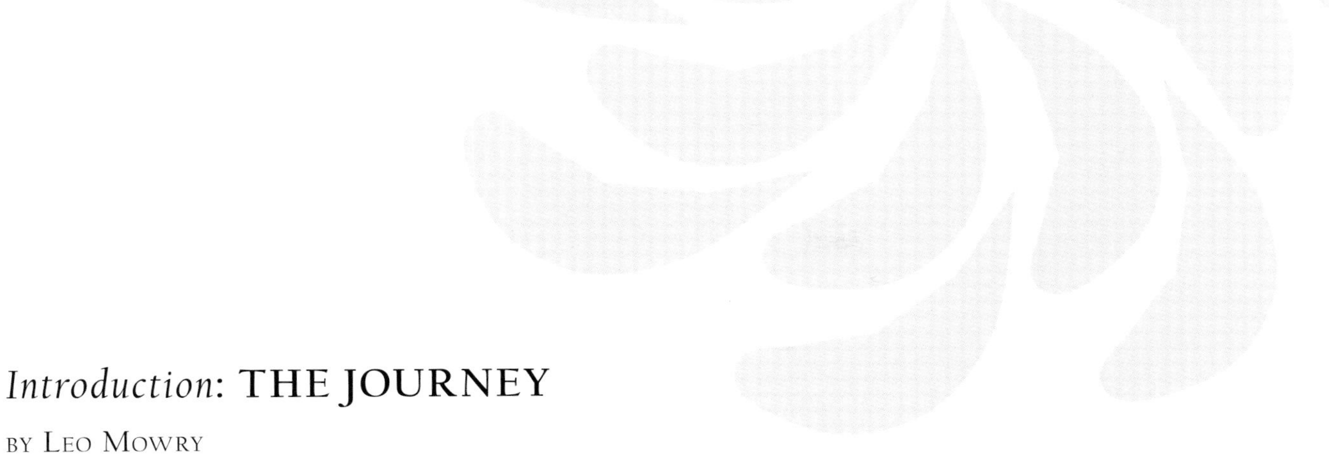

Introduction: THE JOURNEY

BY LEO MOWRY

Susi and I met through a mutual friend who had recommended we get in touch regarding hosting Susi's workshops in Toronto. Our conversation was all business as we discussed the proposed marketing plan, logistics, and what we would each contribute to the venture. Our connection was immediate as we recognized similarities in each other and genuinely enjoyed our time together. The deal was struck. I was hired to handle all the workshop logistics and student registrations for Susi's first **Anatomy & Asana** workshop in Toronto. At the time, I had no idea how profoundly this meeting would change my life.

I was not only the event manager for that first workshop, but also an eager participant. Over the course of that weekend, something shifted inside me. Somehow I knew that my approach to teaching yoga had changed forever.

At the time, I was teaching a lot of vinyasa classes to beginners and more advanced students, and my intention in participating in Susi's workshop was to help me better understand how to keep my students safe in their practices. During the workshop with Susi, however, troubling questions arose. How could I keep teaching as I teach, with the new knowledge that many of my students shouldn't be practicing certain "common" poses like Downward Facing Dog, given the lack of mobility in their shoulders? How could I properly prepare my students' bodies for poses that I now recognized as too advanced for many of them, without compromising the fluidity of a vinyasa practice? Moreover, how would I ensure that my faculty members and I keep every one of our students safe, considering their vastly differing physical realities?

I didn't yet have the answers to these questions. I did, however, have a new toolbox replete with powerful but subtle stabilizing and mobilizing poses, a basic knowledge of proper anatomical alignment, and a few easy principles to which to adhere, thanks to having attended the workshop. I began to teach Susi's principles of creating ease in the body, and use the poses and techniques I had learned in the warm-up and cool-down phases of my classes. My passion for therapeutics flourished.

The way I taught yoga changed dramatically after my first training with Susi. Faculty members at my studio (many of whom by now have also trained with Susi!) began to share the principles of ease and pain-free movement with our students. In our quarterly faculty meetings, I emphasized the basic anatomically-correct foundations that every one of our students must be taught, and we explored, and continue to explore, the myriad of therapeutic techniques.

In 2007, I completed Susi's "The Therapeutic Yoga Intensive". As I've learned to expect when training with Susi, yet another dramatic shift occurred. I realized that to teach from my inner truth, I would have to veer completely away from vinyasa and move into an entirely therapeutics-based teaching approach.

Now a new question arose. How do I continue to teach my advanced-level class and keep them engaged with therapeutics?

I decided to teach my advanced class how therapeutic yoga affects advanced yoga postures. Each class would have a theme — the posture of the day — whether Downward Facing Dog, Triangle, etc. My intention for the class was multi-faceted. By exploring the effects of different therapeutic techniques and principles, the students would:

- Learn and embody the principles of ease
- Understand how subtle movement can dramatically alter their experience of the advanced postures
- Explore new ways of stabilizing and mobilizing, and consequently learn which parts of their bodies require greater stability and mobility
- Develop more self-awareness and understanding of their bodies, and mindfulness and focus in the yoga practice
- Discover an overall sense of ease and groundedness in the poses and the understanding that these qualities are the very essence of yoga

The week after completing "The Therapeutic Yoga Intensive", I began my new experiment. I prepared the students for the dramatic format shift by sharing my intentions with them and letting them know that this was an experiment; that as my knowledge grows, so too does my need to integrate new knowledge into the way I teach. I also let them know how important they are to me, and invited them to share their feedback — positive and negative — with me along the journey.

I knew that in shifting my teaching method, I risked losing some of the students who love vinyasa and who love consistently working hard. Anticipating some dissention in the group, I explained that becoming a more advanced student isn't just about becoming stronger and more flexible. It's also about cultivating the ability to be truly present in the poses; observing, feeling, and being present to the breath and the sensations that arise, as they arise. I explained that one of the pitfalls of becoming an advanced student is that sometimes these important fundamentals are forgotten in exchange for the ambition to accomplish really cool-looking, advanced poses.

I asked the students to return to pure observation and rein in their ambition. I asked for their trust and willingness to explore a new way of approaching the practice, if only for a little while. I added the positive messages that I strongly suspected this new approach would dramatically improve their ability to experience their bodies, and ultimately propel them more quickly, effectively, and safely toward the advanced poses that they so wanted to practice. Each student agreed, but were a little surprised. I don't often begin class with a speech.

The experiment was and continues to be a resounding success! The students were amazed and delighted to discover new things about their bodies that have improved their ability to move in class, and in their daily lives. The opportunity to slow down clearly illustrated physical realities that were impeding progress. For example, one student discovered that side-bending profoundly improved the mobility of her shoulders. Another discovered that stretching the quadriceps improved her ability and comfort in Ustrasana. Every class led to new discoveries that empower the students and led them to greater self-awareness. One day, after bringing the class out of Savasana, one of my long-time students looked at me with shining eyes, shaking her head slowly in wonder, and said: "It just keeps getting better and better". The feedback has been resoundingly positive, and now, months later, the experiment has become the norm.

It has been more than two years since I first joined Susi on this journey into therapeutic applications of yoga, and she and I have now successfully co-produced 8 Toronto workshops focused on yoga therapy. I've completed 86 hours of training with Susi and assist her in her workshops at the annual "Yoga: The Conference and Show" in Toronto. To say that my experience with this new approach has been life-changing would be an understatement.

Not long after I started teaching this new therapeutic approach, I had an opportunity to speak with Susi on the phone. Now close friends, as well as trusted colleagues, I started waxing poetic about this "new" approach: how much the students were learning about themselves and the poses, how incredibly good they felt during and after class, and how much I love what I'm doing!

There was a pause.

"Maybe we should write a book", Susi said.

Flabbergasted and temporarily unable to speak or understand English, I think I sputtered: "Huh?"

"It's time to share this information with others who want to feel stronger and more at ease," Susi added.

I suspect that we continued to chat and managed to wrap up the conversation normally. I don't actually remember. I was numb with shock and joy and fear and excitement, and everything else you might expect to experience when your professional mentor, the person you respect and learn from, and whose teachings have changed your fundamental approach to your way of being, asks you to collaborate on a book. I believe my exact, eloquent words to my partner after getting off the phone were: "Holy Sh#@!"

Leo Mowry
April 2008

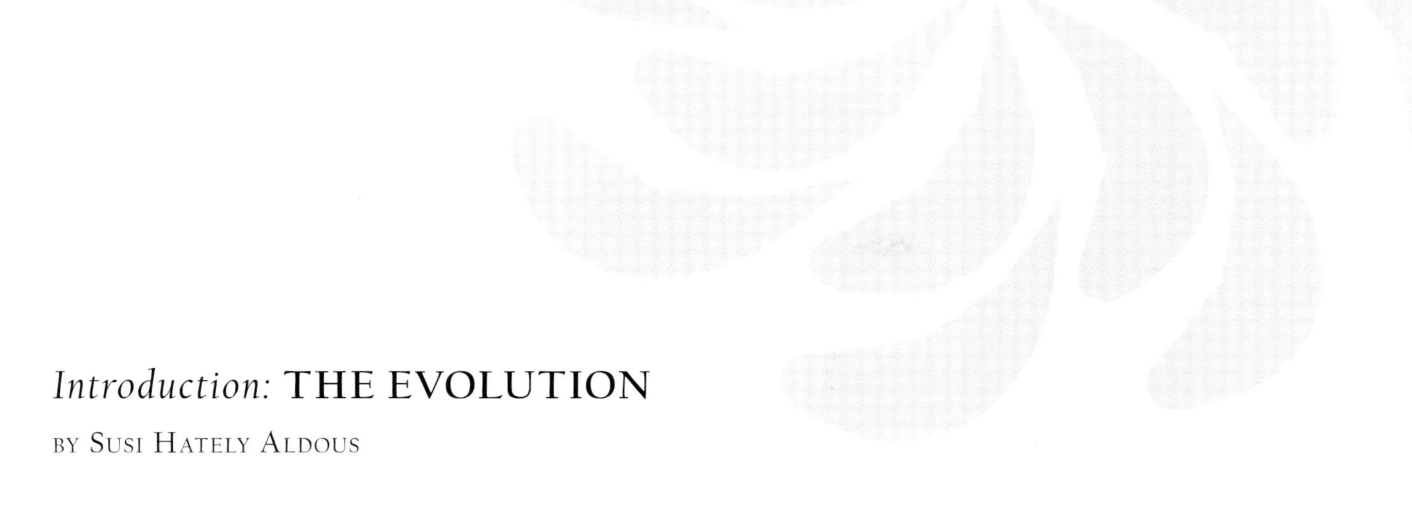

Introduction: THE EVOLUTION

BY SUSI HATELY ALDOUS

Shortly after I graduated from the University of Victoria's Kinesiology program, I worked with physiotherapists and occupational therapists in a variety of rehabilitation settings. My role was to create exercise programs for people who had been injured or had long-standing chronic pain.

In and around that time frame I had stumbled into yoga. I had developed long-standing pain from a variety of athletic pursuits and I seemed to injury myself with each new activity I took on whether it be swimming, running, cycling, hiking. I was in a frustrating state of disrepair.

It was my roommate who suggested yoga to me, and, to be honest, I wasn't all that eager. Nonetheless, something within spoke louder and the following week I was in a class.

I can still remember that class vividly and the moment that the "lights" came on. I knew that yoga would be my ticket out of pain and into something that was stronger, more free. I had no idea how, I just knew.

As the weeks progressed I started to integrate what I was learning into the programs I was creating for my clients. They started to get better faster with the integration of yoga with traditional exercise therapy. I was ecstatic. While I knew that there was much more to yoga, the results of my clients had sucked me in . . . hook, line, and sinker.

As for my own wellbeing, something continued to happen for me too. I remember the day I decided to go for a "one block run", which in total lasted five minutes. Very slowly, I progressively increased my distance, following just one rule — in order to increase my distance, I had to be easily breathing and experiencing no pain. In my mind, it worked — I ran the Vancouver 10 K Sun Run four months later absolutely pain-free.

Shortly thereafter, I moved to Calgary. I continued my yoga practice and began studying to be a yoga teacher. A year or so later, when I began to teach my first yoga classes, I looked into the sea of faces and wondered — now what? All I could see were a cornucopia of tight and hyperflexible bodies. I was supposed to teach them Level 1 Yoga and all I could wonder was, "How on earth am I going to teach all of these people who are all so unbalanced?"

The year was 1999 — the dawn of applying my anatomical knowledge to yoga. I began to focus in on specific joint movement, building mobility and stability of each joint. When I was satisfied with what I saw unwinding and unfolding, I then started to teach the classic asanas. Students loved my approach, and my classes were always very full. Students were feeling good, their athletic performance improved, and their pain levels dropped.

And then something interesting started to happen. More and more people who were experiencing chronic pain started to come to class. Physiotherapists began to refer patients to my classes. Physicians, massage therapists and chiropractors began to refer their patients. These medical professionals and body workers had heard about my approach, had seen the results in their own clients, and saw it as a very viable way for improving the health and wellbeing of their clientele.

My teaching morphed again. The variety of people within my classes was so great — people with back pain, repetitive strain, chronic pain, people who had recently recovered from pain, triathletes who wanted to experience a "best race" — I couldn't just teach one style of class. So I began to customize my teaching and my classes.

I designed custom programs for each person in the group. With this style of teaching, people could continue to expand and grow at their own pace, and when they got out of pain, they could continue to strengthen, stabilize and unwind their issues and gain better function. The beauty of this type of teaching is that each person was able to feel within. They could "get real" about where they were on any given day and from that place build their practice, find ease, and create lightness. I still teach this way today — I call it **Customized Yoga Therapy**.

Many of my clients come to see me when they are very much in pain, and continue to learn from me when they are well out of pain, so I continue to teach a spectrum of people with a variety of needs. For all of them, their premise for learning from me is the same — to deepen their function and their abilities. You may be thinking — how can you address such a wide spectrum of ability and function? There is one thing that is consistent. Whether someone is in pain and is learning how to get out of pain, or whether someone has learned how to be out of pain and is now building more strength and ease, my fundamental belief in building functional and balanced movement is that you need to build mobility that is balanced with stability, strength that is balanced with softness, and all movements must occur in a pain-free range.

In working with me, all of my clients have come to learn that their bodies are "plastic", that change can occur. They have learned that they just need to tap into the specific stimulus to help them make that change. My job is to help them with that stimulus, and that is the foundation of the **Customized Yoga Therapy** program.

So when Leo called me back in the Fall of 2007 to wax poetically about her new approach to teaching, I knew that she had stumbled upon a deeper level of understanding of balance, ease, strength, mobility and stability. I knew that she had applied the **Anatomy and Asana** principles in a way that could serve a vast number of people who wanted to gain greater ease and balance. I knew that this was information that needed to be shared with other yoga students and teachers so that they too could begin to experience this transformation.

This book will benefit you particularly if:

You are a yoga student who:

- wants to deepen your awareness, strength, and mobility of your body while in yoga asanas . . .
- wants to improve your level of functioning and if you are in pain, how to get out of pain in a long-lasting way . . .
- wants to be able to perform your other activities with greater ease, strength, and power . . .

And/or

You are a yoga teacher who:

- has been impacted by the principles and techniques of **Anatomy and Asana**, and you want to integrate them into your regular yoga classes but aren't sure how . . .

- has been teaching your students therapeutically and are not sure how to take them to the next level, to engage them more fully, evoking greater strength and stability, all the while deepening their sense of ease . . .

- has a feeling of limitation or "stuckness" that you intuitively feel can be shifted but you aren't sure where or how to explore . . .

. . . this book will give you plenty of ideas and techniques to expand your practice.

The beauty of what you are about to read is that it is based on fundamental anatomical and movement principles, outlined in both layperson's and anatomical language. Leo does not have a degree in Kinesiology but she has plenty of training with me and has worked intently with the principles of **Anatomy and Asana**. Together, Leo and I have blended my anatomical and biomechanical knowledge and yoga teaching expertise with her knowledge and expertise and we have spanned a vast spectrum for understanding movement, anatomy, awareness, and observation. No matter where you are at in your movement education, this book will serve you.

For some of you who pick up this book, what we are offering here may represent a radical shift in your perception of the practice, and you may ask yourself whether or not this is a good thing. As I see it, the proof of the pudding is in the eating . . . our collective students love what they are learning. They have experienced and understand that *"it doesn't matter what age you are, your body can unwind, gain strength, move without pain and gain functioning"*. Our students feel younger, stronger, and more at ease. What could be better than that?

HOW THIS BOOK IS LAID OUT:

In Part I of this book, Leo will describe how to use the 7-week curriculum that we have developed for **Advancing Your Yoga Practice: The Art of Slowing Down**. Part II provides a review of the **Principles of Anatomy and Asana**. These are the foundational principles that have guided my personal practice and my teaching since day one. Part III is the curriculum itself. For those practitioners and teachers who have not had formal anatomy and physiology training, we have included anatomical representations that you can reference to deepen your understanding as we move through the curriculum. Within each session Leo and I will take you through step by step — clearly outlining the intention and purpose of each posture or exercise, along with a review of the anatomical considerations for each posture.

Leo and I had much fun pulling this together and I believe that you will receive information and ideas that you can immediately apply in your personal practice, whether as a student or a teacher.

Happy exploring,

Susi Hately Aldous
April 2008

Part I - THE CURRICULUM

The curriculum in this book includes seven unique yoga classes. Although many of the techniques explored in these classes are suitable for beginners, the classes are designed for advanced students who have experienced the poses once before. By advanced we mean a higher degree of connection and body awareness, which tends to be present in a more experienced yoga practitioner.

Unlike with most yoga classes, these sequences begin with practicing the "theme pose", before the opening relaxation. The assumption is that you are familiar with the "theme poses" and can get into them safely without risking injury. The opening relaxation poses were selected to create mobility and ease in a way that will affect your experience in the "theme poses".

Thus, the "theme poses" are practiced periodically throughout the sequences, so that you can compare how you feel in the pose after practicing the various types of therapeutic mobilizing and stabilizing techniques. Hopefully, by the end of each sequence, you will feel a vastly improved sense of ease in the poses and feel more comfortable in your own body.

We recommend asking yourself how you feel throughout each sequence. This will lead you to greater self-awareness and promote self-inquiry. The feedback we most often hear are words like: longer, easier, more fluid, connected, stronger, etc.

If you have experienced **Anatomy and Asana** training with Susi, you have learned that there is no precise "recipe" for creating proper alignment. As each human body is different, so too is its stabilizing and mobilizing needs. The methodology in this series of sequences is based on what type of stabilizing and opening bodies typically need to practice the "theme poses" comfortably and in a balanced way.

In practicing these sequences yourself or as a teacher teaching them to your students, however, you might observe that certain people need more of a different kind of mobility or stability to effectively practice the poses. Use the information offered here to guide you as you experiment with using different techniques in different sequences. You'll undoubtedly discover that most of the techniques incorporated into the specific "theme" sequences have a lot of value for many other poses, too!

Finally, at the foundation of these sequences are the basic principles of creating ease, thereby improving mobility, stability and reducing or eliminating pain. These principles are:

NO PAIN ALLOWED. NOT EVEN A LITTLE BIT. We encourage you to work within your pain-free range of motion. When pain happens, tension results and the potential for ease in movement is eliminated. This absolutely counteracts our purpose. A pain-free range of motion engenders effective healing, and increased mobility and stability. An "in-pain" range of motion does the opposite.

NATURAL BREATH. By cultivating a natural breath you create greater relaxation. Sometimes, even with common breath techniques like Ujjayi or Three-Part Breath, striving occurs. A forced breath, as opposed to an easy breath, creates inappropriate tension. Be cognizant that you aren't overdoing a more complicated breath technique.

The breath is also a key indicator of whether you are working too hard. If you cannot breathe easily in a pose, you've gone beyond your "edge".

NO CLICKING IN THE JOINTS. Clicking implies an opportunity for better function — something is not moving as functionally as it could. You're trying to create space, not force it! By moving in a "click-free" range of motion, you actually increase your "click-free" range of motion. By allowing yourself to continually click in the joints, you dramatically reduce the potential for creating more space in the joints and the resulting ease of movement.

As you begin to apply this knowledge to your practice, the main thing to bear in mind is that at the core of this practice is the intention of creating ease. If there is pain, forced breath, clicking, striving, struggling, or tension of any kind, you simply cannot create the ease that should be the foundation of every healing yoga practice.

Part II – PRINCIPLES OF MOVEMENT

Susi Hately Aldous

The basis for the yoga practices offered in this book, whether for a student or teacher, revolves around **Anatomy and Asana's** eight principles of movement. Found in the fields of body mechanics, movement science, physiology, and anatomy, when you understand these principles and couple them with your knowledge of muscle function and movement, your practice changes — you'll be more aware, you'll be stronger, and you'll experience more freedom.

Let's take a look:

Do not think of these eight principles as a linear list where you begin with one and continue with the next. Rather, each impacts and is impacted by the rest — much like a series of eight conjoining circles.

Our life is an apprenticeship to the truth that around every circle another can be drawn; that there is no end in nature, but every end is a beginning, and under every deep a lower deep opens. —Ralph Waldo Emerson

1. NOURISH RELAXATION.

Relaxation is a time for coming into yourself, of getting in touch with how you were with your day and how your day was with you. It enables you to tap into your flow and to set a baseline from which you can work — careful to not get ahead of yourself while staying diligent in unwinding muscle and fascia, tapping into and connecting to who and what you are.

It's also a time to become aware of your breath. Notice how your inhale and exhale are moving. Are you having to concentrate in order to relax; are you able to feel where the breath is moving in your body and where your body isn't as accepting (for example, some people feel their breath easily in their belly but not so much in their upper rib cage, for others it is the opposite)? Are you able to just watch the breath, or are you trying to change it?

Allow your practice to honour these moments where your body is letting you know about its energy reserves, its ability to breathe, and its ability to settle and be still.

2. BEGIN WITH THE SPINE IN MIND.
Once settled in body and breath you can begin to move.

The spine is the central hub from which all movement occurs. At its essence, the spine is a collection of bones, muscles, fascia, blood, lymph, and nerve vessels. When tight and imbalanced, the spine will impact shoulder and hip range of motion; it will impact your ability to twist, bend, and move upside down. And, more specifically, if the superficial spinal muscles are tight and short, and the deeper spinal muscles are weak, you may feel a mishmash of symptoms, limitations, pulls, and twangs in your shoulders, elbows, wrists, and/or knees. Even before you initiate any movement in the body, consider how the intended movement will impact the spine and in particular what range of motion is available within the spine.

3. CONNECT SPINAL MOVEMENT WITH MOVEMENT AT YOUR LARGEST JOINTS FIRST.
Once your body is relaxed and you are able to feel the spine as the place from which movement radiates, the next intention is to enable free and easy movement of the limbs. The simplest way to create this is by focusing on the largest joints first, specifically the shoulder and hip joints. This may be surprising for some yogis since there are particular systems that build the poses from the hands and feet.

From an anatomical perspective the hip and shoulder joints are more proximal, or closer to, the spine than the hands and feet, making it easier to maintain awareness while releasing inappropriate tension or creating better stability.

4. MOVE JOINTS IN THEIR OPTIMUM RANGE OF MOTION.
This is where you get to choose. What is optimal for you? Do you have osteoarthritis or bursitis? Does one joint move more smoothly and easily through its range of motion than another? Find the degree of motion where you are feeling at ease, you can breathe, the joint is moving in the direction it was designed to move in, and you feel no pain.

5. DEVELOP CORE STABILITY: BOOST UP YOUR BANDHAS AND BREATHE.
Core stability is the "Steady Eddy" of our practices. It keeps us solid, unwavering, and fluid, as well as enabling us to respond to the twists and turns, the increases and decreases in tempo and rhythm. The result — we stand taller, we breathe easier, and our backs, hips, and knees feel so much better.

To define core stability, I really like using the following description: core stability is a balance between mobility and strength – the balance of strong core muscles found along the midline of the body from the base of the skull to the bottom of the feet, combined with the freedom of movement at the hip, shoulder, and vertebral joints as well as at the elbow, wrist, knee, and ankle joints. Without this balance, the body will be either too rigid (too much strength and too little mobility) or limp and spiritless (too much mobility with too little strength).

So to distinguish what the core is we need to look at several muscles. Beginning from the feet, these are:

- Peroneus Longus and Tibialis Posterior
- Hip Adductors
- Pelvic Floor

These muscles balance with the:

- Hip Abductors and External Rotators
- Transversus Abdominis
- Multifidi

Which work together with the:

- Deep Flexors of the neck

The following muscles support our level of core stability because they help stabilize the shoulder girdle:

- Pectoralis Minor
- Trapezius
- Rhomboids
- Serratus Anterior

In yoga, the stability in our core enables us to go from fast to slow, and slow to fast, and it also gives us the strength and ease to stay in an asana for an extended period of time. To fully reap the benefits of the core, we have to blend it with breath. If breath isn't fluid and free the core will not be supple and strong. So enjoy the ease and settle into strength.

6. ADOPT RELAXED RESILIENCE.
This is where depth in your yoga practice is developed. Relaxation occurs in layers, beginning with breath and continuing with awareness. Layer by layer, you will develop more awareness. With more awareness, you'll be better able to perceive levels of tension and freedom that exist in your body. This is what I call "depth". Imagine this: You are halfway through a class, and you are feeling tired or distracted. Reconnect by noticing where and how you are breathing. Try not to change it — just notice it and practice there. See what happens.

7. BE GENEROUS WITH YOURSELF: MOVE IN YOUR *PAIN-FREE* RANGE OF MOTION.
Ahh . . . the loaded word ***pain***. What it means to one person could mean something entirely different to another. For clarity, consider a spectrum of pain: good pain consists of muscle fatigue, the point at which the muscle fibres can no longer contract. The nerve fibres keep sending stimulating signals, but the muscles aren't responding, either because their energy reserves are exhausted or there is a buildup of lactic acid. On the other side of the spectrum is the bad pain that burns, strains, rips, and tears.

It is the pain that causes your brow to furrow, your teeth to clench, your breath to be held, and your body to reverberate with tension.

If you take a moment and move only in your pain-free range of motion, you will notice that not only does your range improve, it improves faster and continues to be pain-free!

Why does this work? When we move in an "in-pain" range of motion, we increase tightness and tension in our bodies. With increased tension unwinding can't occur, and the issue that is creating the pain doesn't get resolved.

So, breathe, move a little more slowly, be aware, and stay in your pain-free range of motion.

8. LESS IS MORE: DEVELOP STRENGTH, STABILITY, MOBILITY, AND FLEXIBILITY IN THE SIMPLE YOGA ASANAS BEFORE MOVING INTO THE COMPLEX YOGA ASANAS.

A simple yoga asana is one which requires fewer joint motions. For example Tadasana is simple. Vrksasana (Tree Pose) is more complex because now one hip is doing one motion while the other hip is doing a different set of motions.

Another example is Dandasana (Staff Pose), which is simpler than Marichyasana (Pose Dedicated to the Sage Marichi). In Dandasana, both legs are doing the same thing at their respective hip joints. Balance is straightforward to create. With Marichyasana there are two different leg positions and a twist has been added. The arms are being used to support the twist. Since more is going on there is greater complexity. With more complexity there is greater potential for strain or injury.

The key then, is to start small, take baby steps, and bite off no more than you can chew. Gain the mobility, stability, strength and ease in the simple asanas before moving into the complex asanas.

Now that the principles of movement have been explored, let's move into the practice.

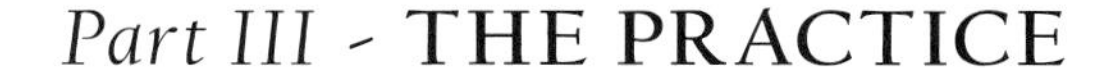

Part III - THE PRACTICE

The following seven weeks of practice evolved out of the principles of **Anatomy and Asana** and Therapeutic Yoga when applied to classic yoga asanas. The intent behind each of the sequences is to give you more freedom, strength and ease and less pain, tightness and tension.

Students who practice in this way have developed greater body awareness, less pain, and better function. To help you along in that direction consider the following:

As you practice remain humble. Allow yourself to explore the asanas and the movements. Allow yourself to notice what is there — does it feel good, can I breathe, what does this tightness feel like, how does this release compare to the release on the other side? Remain curious of how your body is responding, all the while staying in your pain-free, click-free, and easy breathing range of motion. While these practices have helped many people, and are based on long standing anatomical principles, your bodymind is your bodymind. If something doesn't work for you, we encourage you to ease out of the pose.

If you are a teacher and you are taking these sequences into your class, encourage your students to explore and to feel. If you are a teacher, know that there is as much for you to learn from your students as you have to share as their teacher. Be humble, give space, and breathe. Enjoy the transformations.

A SPECIAL NOTE: THE ORDER OF THIS CURRICULUM

This series begins with **Adho Mukha Svanasana (Downward Facing Dog)** since in this pose, many people experience inappropriate tension and/or hyperextension. There are many questions around this asana, which is why the curriculum begins here.

Trikonasana (Triangle) is next because the ability to not side-bend in some students is problematic and can easily be resolved with isolating where the tightness or imbalance resides in individual bodies. By resolving that, Trikonasana can evolve and blossom.

Parivritta Trikonasana (Revolved Triangle) is a natural progression from Trikonasana.

Uttanasana (Standing Forward Bend) is a fundamental standing pose and is a logical precursor to **Virabhadrasana I and II (Warrior I and II).**

Ustrasana comes last since so many people have trouble with more advanced backbends. With several weeks of prepratory therapeutic movement, the hope is there is more awareness, openness, stability and strength to explore this asana.

As you explore these sequences in your own practice as a student and/or teacher, focus on how the movements feel. If you would like to share your insights, please email us at **iloveanatomy@anatomyandasana.com**.

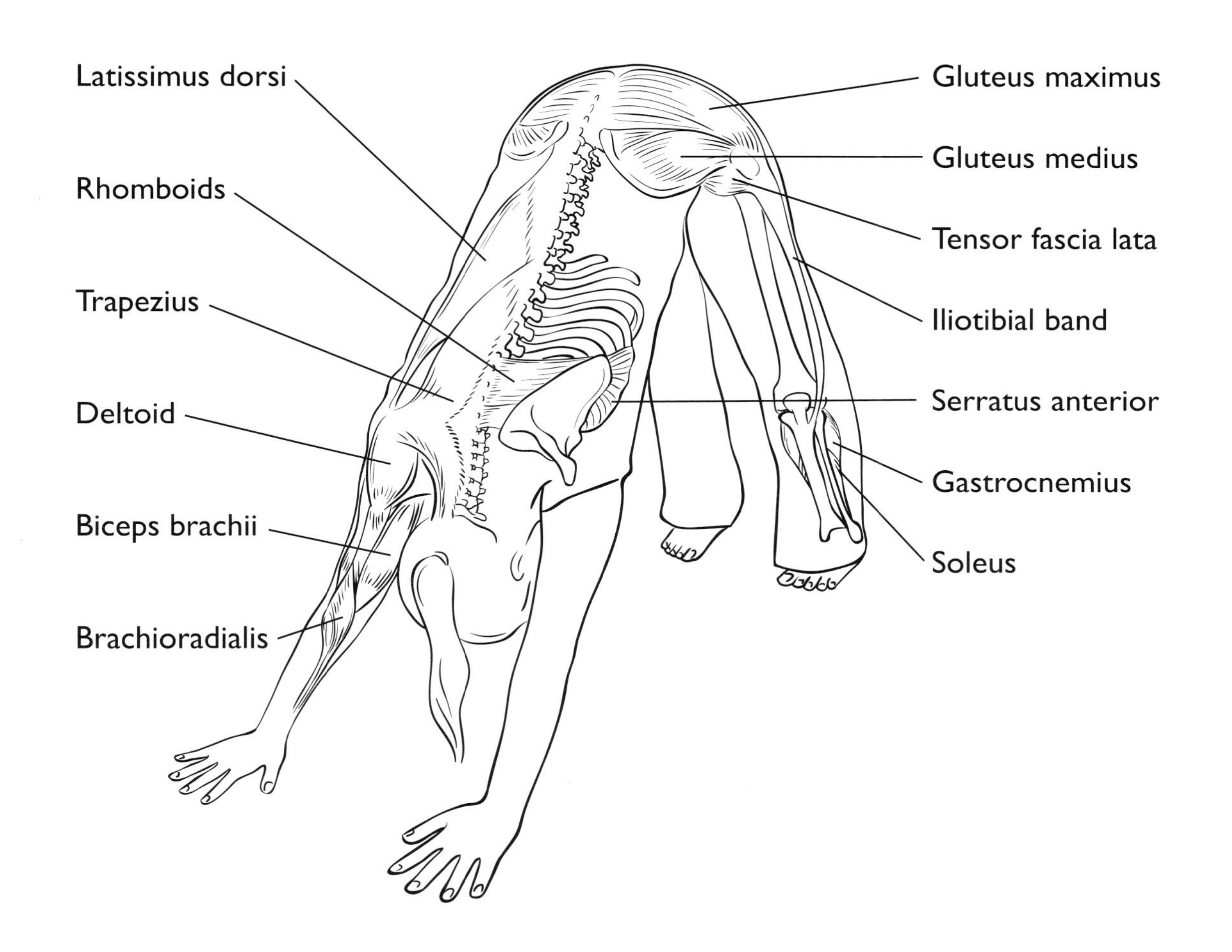

adho mukha svanasana

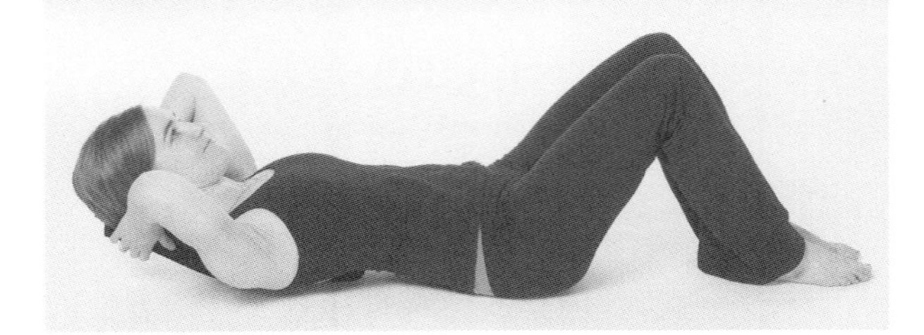

opening relaxation - 2

Adho Mukha Svanasana

(Downward Facing Dog)

Consider your Anatomy: To move safely into Adho Mukha Svanasana, or Downward Facing Dog, a few things need to occur – there needs to be an adequate range of motion and stability in the shoulder and pelvic girdles, without putting too much inappropriate tension through the torso, spine or rib cage. With optimum range of motion and stability, the lines of energy or force are easily transferred to the arms and hands, and to the legs and feet for a stable, restful and strong Dog pose.

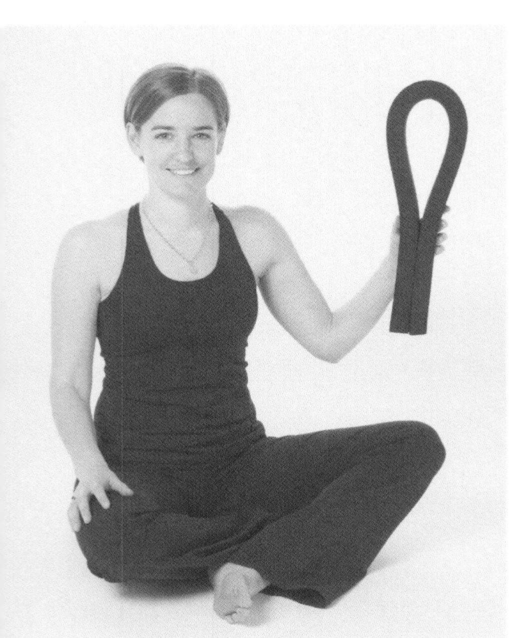

opening relaxation - 1

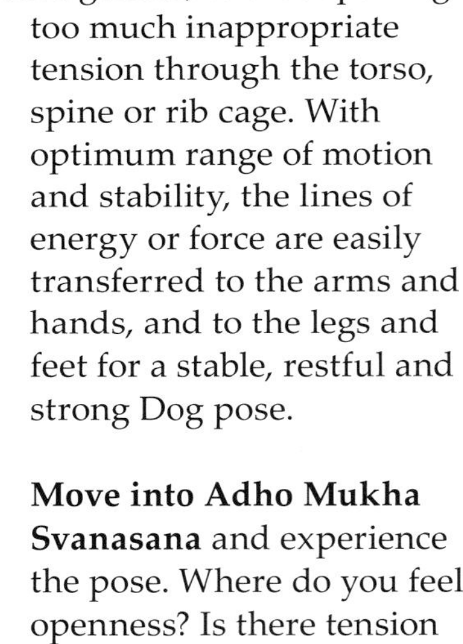

Move into Adho Mukha Svanasana and experience the pose. Where do you feel openness? Is there tension or discomfort? Where? Are you struggling? How?

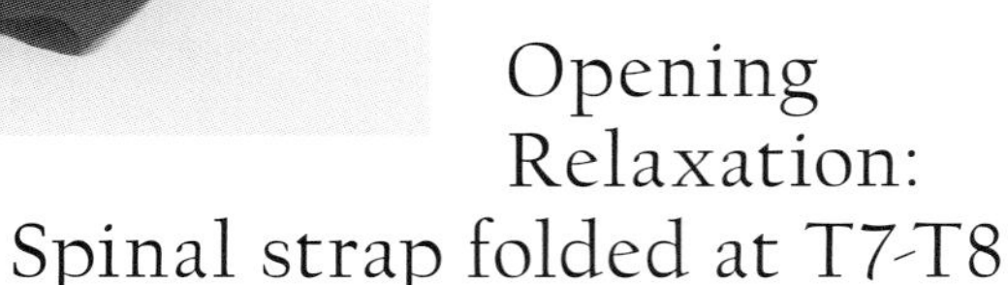

Opening Relaxation: Spinal strap folded at T7-T8

1. Fold a spinal strap in half. Place the bottom of the fold at T7-T8 (where a bra strap would be).

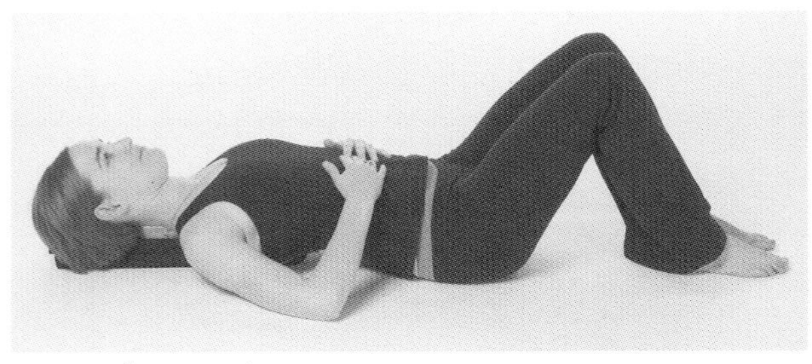

opening relaxation - 3

2. Recline with the knees bent and feet planted on the ground. The spinal strap runs upward along the spine from the fold at T7-T8 and supports the head. If there is discomfort in the back, elevate the buttocks with a folded blanket. Another alternative is to lay on the single strap – i.e. not folded. If you don't have a spinal strap or if the sensations caused by the pose are too intense, place a rolled yoga mat in the same position at T7-T8.

3. Relax in the position, and observe the sensations that arise. This might not be entirely comfortable! Imagine gently "expanding the chest" (where you have the greatest sensation of openness) as you inhale, and "letting go" as you exhale. I recommend at least five minutes in this pose to allow the body to settle effectively. As in any pose, however, your limit might be reached prior to this. At any point, if pain occurs, the breath becomes haggard, or tension arises that can't be released with the breath and conscious softening, remove the strap.

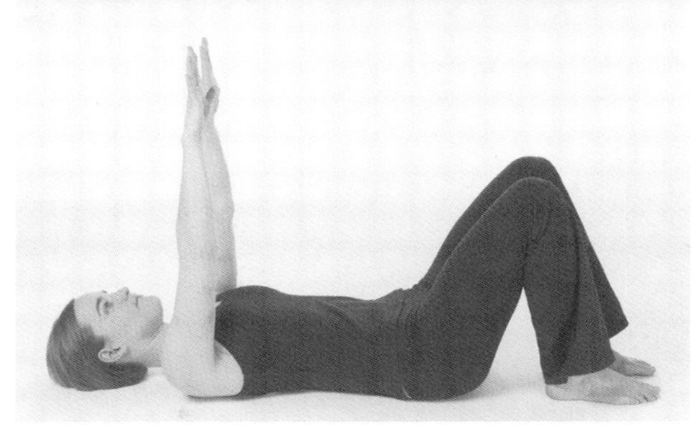

hands to the sky

4. After the allotted time in this pose, remove the spinal strap and return to the reclined position without it. Notice the sensations in the front and back of the upper body. Is there a greater sense of space/openness in the chest? A greater connection of the upper back with the ground? How does it feel?

Reclined Shoulder Mobility

1. Stay in the reclined position. If it's comfortable, the legs can be extended on the mat out in front of you.

2. Touch your thumb-tips together. The following two positions will help to even out the motion between your left and right sides, bringing balance to your shoulder girdle and neck.

Pullovers

(Also known as Hands to Sky)

1. Elevate and straighten the arms so the wrists are directly over the shoulders. The arms are extending straight up toward the sky (not back behind you!).

2. Gently draw the arm bones into the shoulder sockets and bring the shoulder blades down toward the floor. Moving with the breath, begin to slowly reach the arms toward the sky, and then draw them back down again. Repeat 5-10 times.

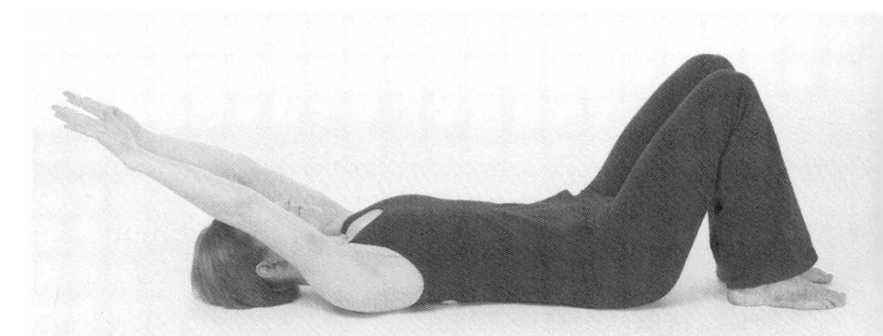

hands and arms overhead

Pullovers

(Also known as Hands and Arms Overhead)

1. With the fingers toward the sky, begin to arc the arms overhead. Be sure to move in a pain-free range of motion. The idea is to allow the arms to move in a half-circle. No matter what the range, the furthest range will be to move alongside the ears (i.e. don't go for the floor). Here are a few conditions to follow in order to gain better motion and function:

• No clicking or pain. Remember, you're trying to create space. If clicking, pain, or general unsteadiness occurs, be sure to shift into your click-free, pain-free and easy range of motion. We know this can be very humbling and challenging! We also know that the range of motion may increase

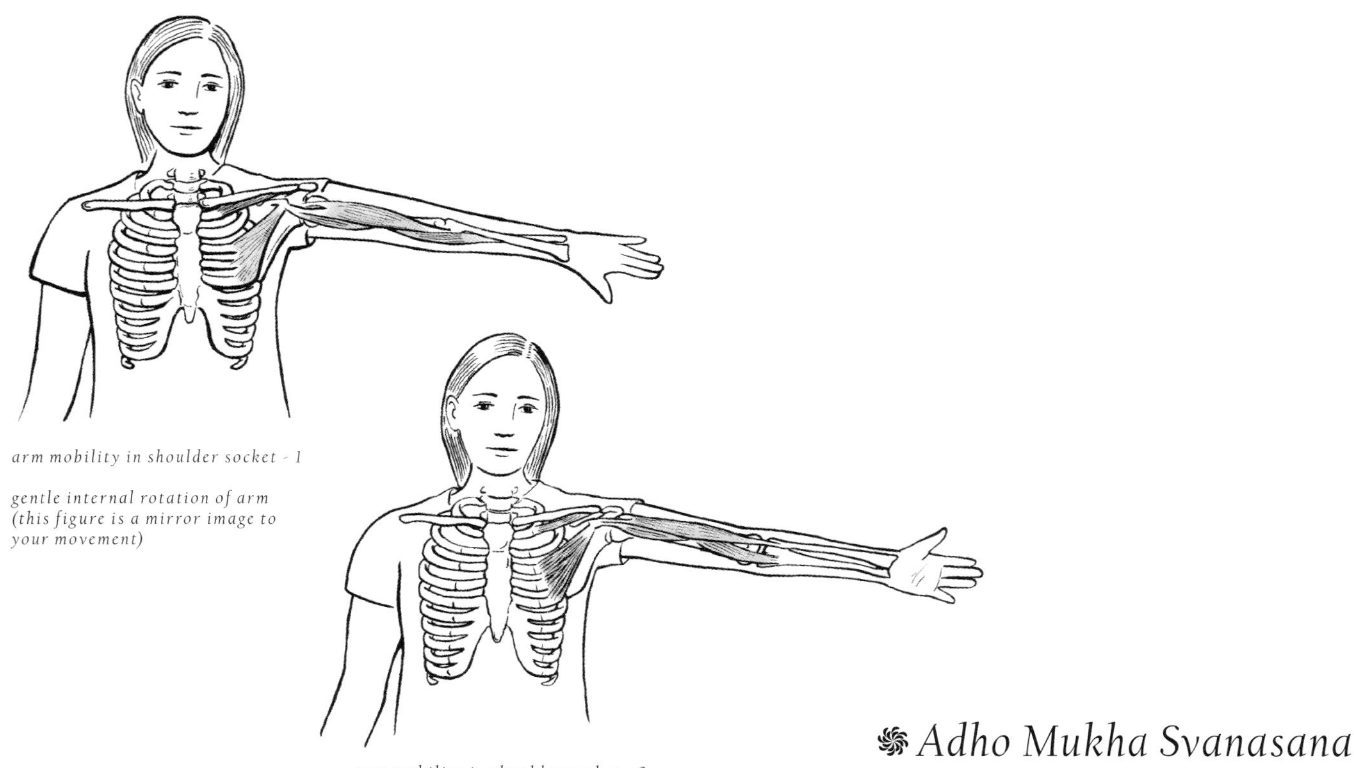

arm mobility in shoulder socket - 1

gentle internal rotation of arm (this figure is a mirror image to your movement)

arm mobility in shoulder socket - 2

gentle external rotation of arm

while practicing this exercise, but only if these guidelines are followed.

• No back bending. If back bending occurs as the arms start to come overhead, the mobility required for the movement to occur is being facilitated by the spine. The objective in this exercise is to create easy mobility of the arm bone in the shoulder socket, not in the spine. The arm arcs should stop before the backbend occurs.

2. Repeat the arm arcs several times.

Adho Mukha Svanasana

Arm Mobility in Shoulder Socket

Come into a comfortable seated position. Relax the shoulders, connect with your sit bones and lengthen through the torso and spine, encouraging space and the spine's natural curves. The arms rest comfortably at the sides of the body.

1. Lift arms slightly so that the fingers/hands don't touch the ground.

2. Keeping the shoulders stable and relaxed, slowly being to rotate the arm bones in the shoulder sockets. This is a very small arm movement. Do your best to keep your shoulder blade from moving. If it does, make the motion smaller. Repeat several times then relax the arms at the sides of the body.

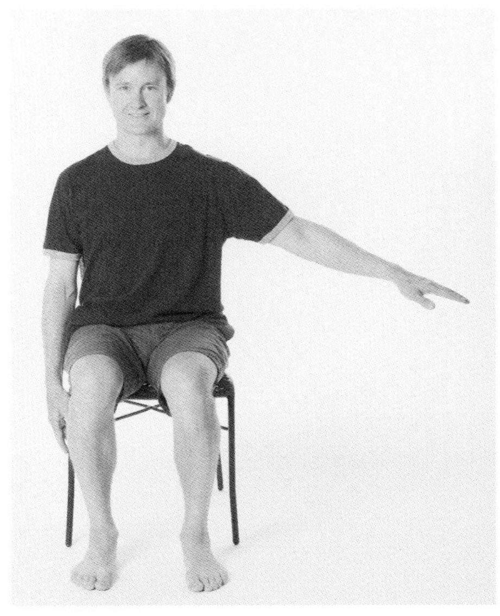

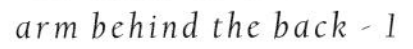

arm behind the back - 1

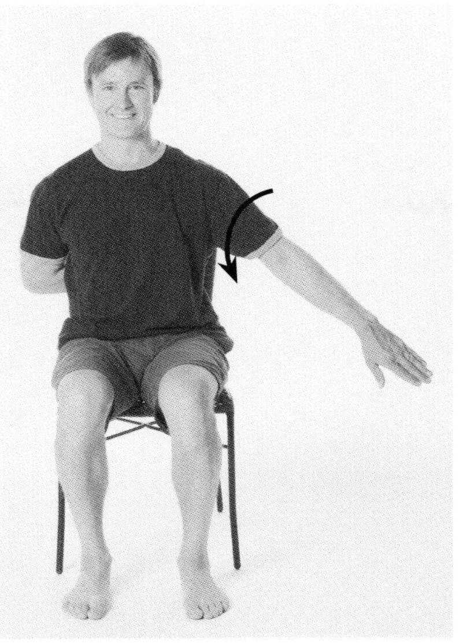

arm behind the back - 2

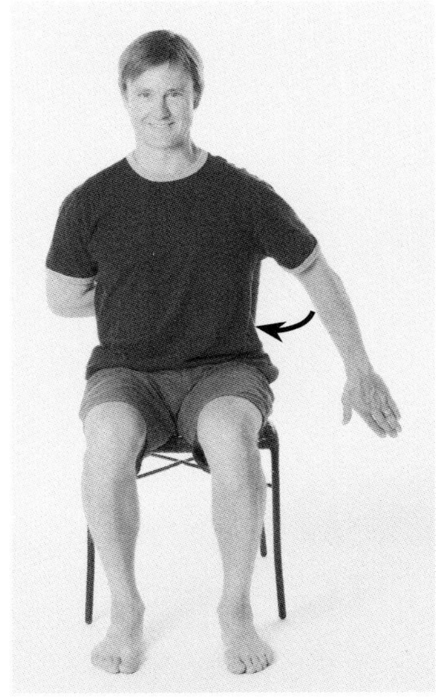

arm behind the back - 3

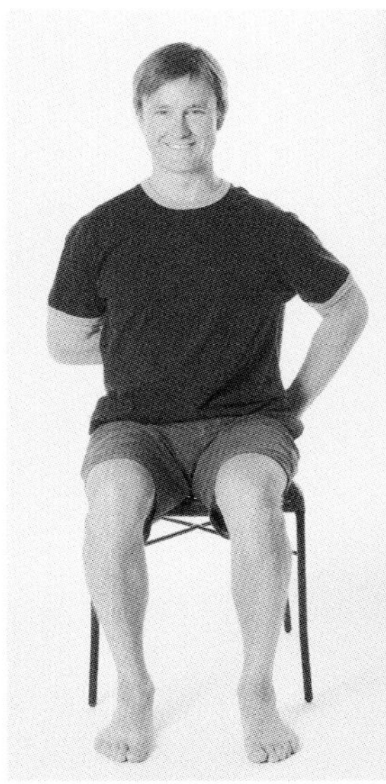

arm behind the back - 4

Arm Behind the Back

1. Lift the left arm slightly out to the left.

2. Internally rotate the arm, and slowly begin to move it behind the body. The elbow will bend.

3. Take several easy breaths in place, noticing the sensations that arise. Relax and change sides. Soften the space between your eyes.

Roll Out Shoulders with Tennis Ball

1. Sit or stand facing away from the wall and place a tennis ball at the upper back.

2. Apply slight pressure and observe what you feel. If you discover places that feel particularly tight, pause in place and smile.

3. Move slowly left and right, up and down, exploring the shoulder and upper back region.

4. Do not place or roll the tennis ball at the spine.

5. When you are finished on one side, pause with both arms relaxed at the sides of the body and notice if there are different sensations in the left and right side.

6. Roll out the other side of the upper back.

7. When complete, pause with both arms relaxed at the sides of the body and notice the sensations.

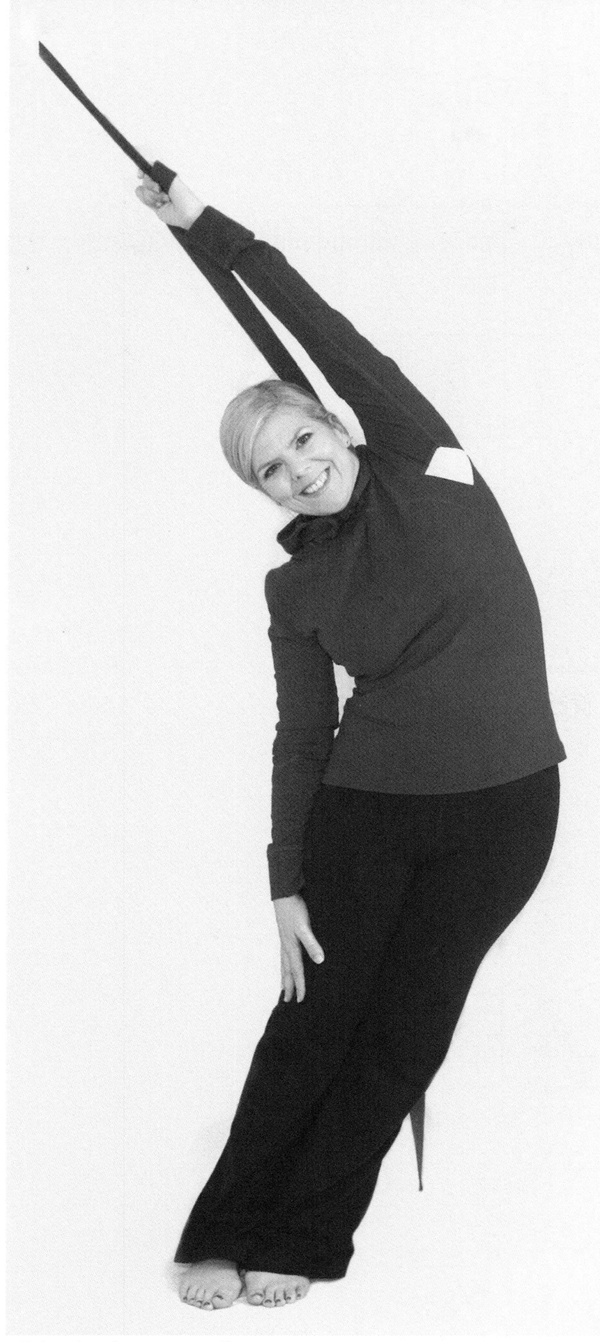

side bend with strap over door

❁ *Adho Mukha Svanasana*

Side Bend with Strap Over Door

1. Place the top end of a strap over the top of a door and close the door, pulling the strap taut. Stand perpendicular to the wall and take the arm that's farthest from the door overhead. Loop the strap around the hand a couple of times until it's stable and the strap won't slide when you pull away from the wall.

2. Holding the strap, start to lean the body away from the door, leading with the hips. Be here for a few breaths, then return to standing.

3. Next, lean away from the door but lead from your ribs. Explore a few more times, leading with the waist or underarm. (The sensations in the side body will probably differ depending on what part of the body presses away from the wall.)

4. The strap can feel tight around the hand. Feel free to pause and relax the hand periodically, if necessary.

5. Release the arm and come into Mountain. Observe the sensations left and right.

Change sides.

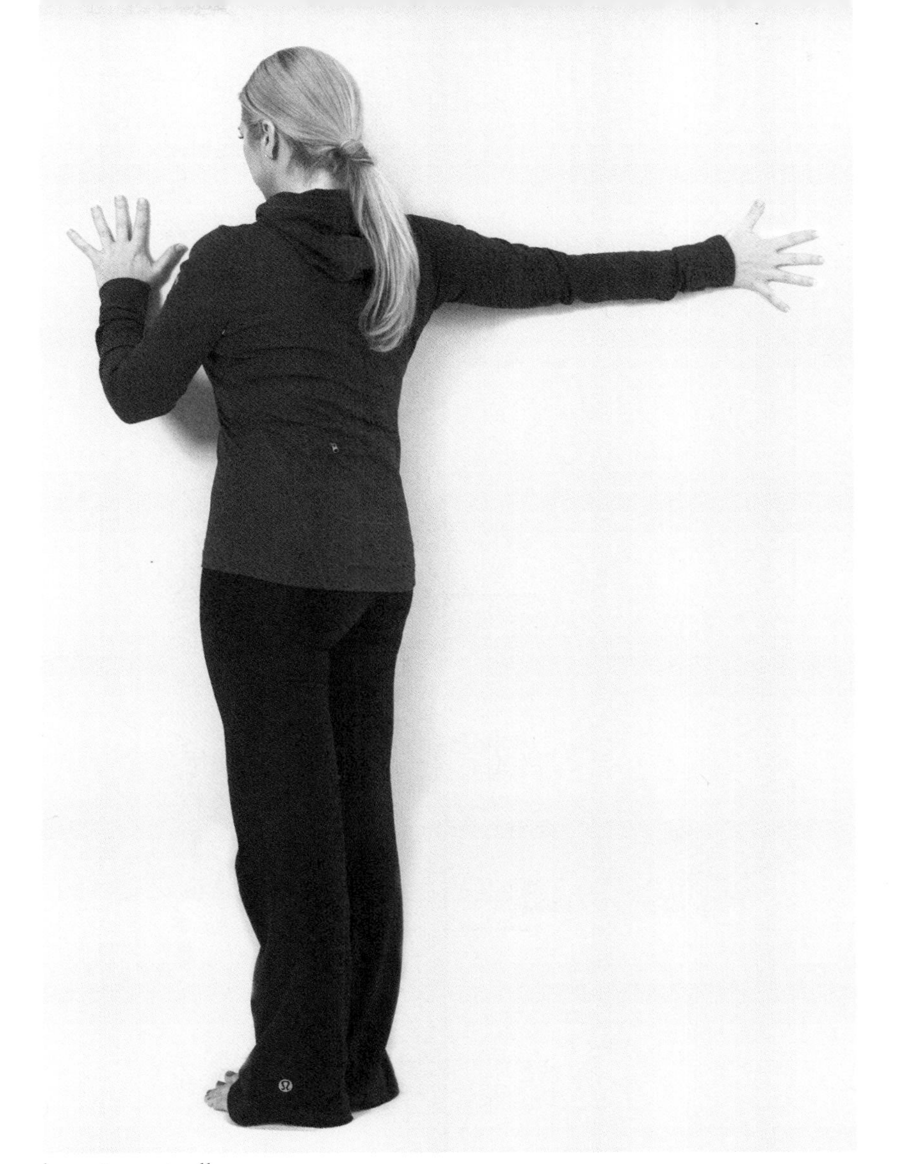

heart opener at wall

Adho Mukha Svanasana

Heart Opener at Wall

1. Stand facing the wall, up against it. Extend the right arm out along the wall at shoulder height. The palm is flat on the wall, fingers spread, and the arm bone is drawing back into the shoulder socket.

2. Notice what you feel. Are there are any sensations of stretching or tightness in the arm, shoulder or chest? If so, stay here and breathe easily and observe the sensations. If there is no stretch sensation, slowly rotate the feet and body away from the outstretched arm. Stop as soon as a stretch is observed. The shoulder should stay relaxed and free of gripping or inappropriate tension. Stay here and breathe easy observing the sensations. If tingling or numbness occur, take a break until it subsides.

3. Lower the arm after a minute or two (assuming there was no pain, tingling or numbness) and stand in Mountain observing the sensations in both the left and right side.

Change sides.

IF YOUR COMPASSION DOES NOT

INCLUDE YOURSELF, IT IS INCOMPLETE.

—*Jack Kornfield*

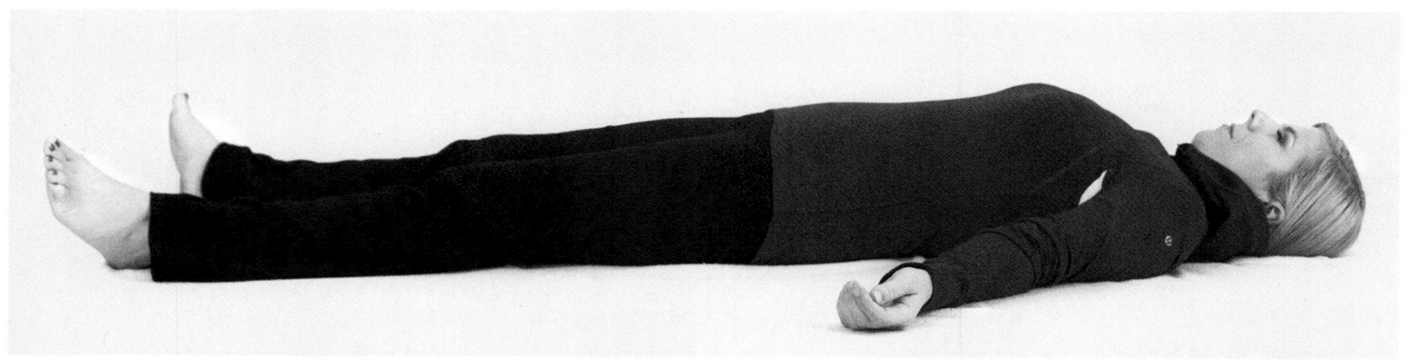

savasana

Adho Mukha Svanasana

Savasana

As you lay back, feel your breath and feel your body. Become aware of your body laying on the floor and how your breath moves your belly on the inhale and exhale.

Questions to consider:
How did my body feel with the black strap? Did I enjoy it, if so why? If not, why not? Am I able to differentiate between the feelings on opposites sides of my body? How does it feel to slow down and focus inward? What differences, subtle or obvious, can I feel in the pose from the first to the last instance? Do I think that I have a better awareness of the movement required to access this pose safely and effectively in my practice? Which exercise had the greatest impact, and why?

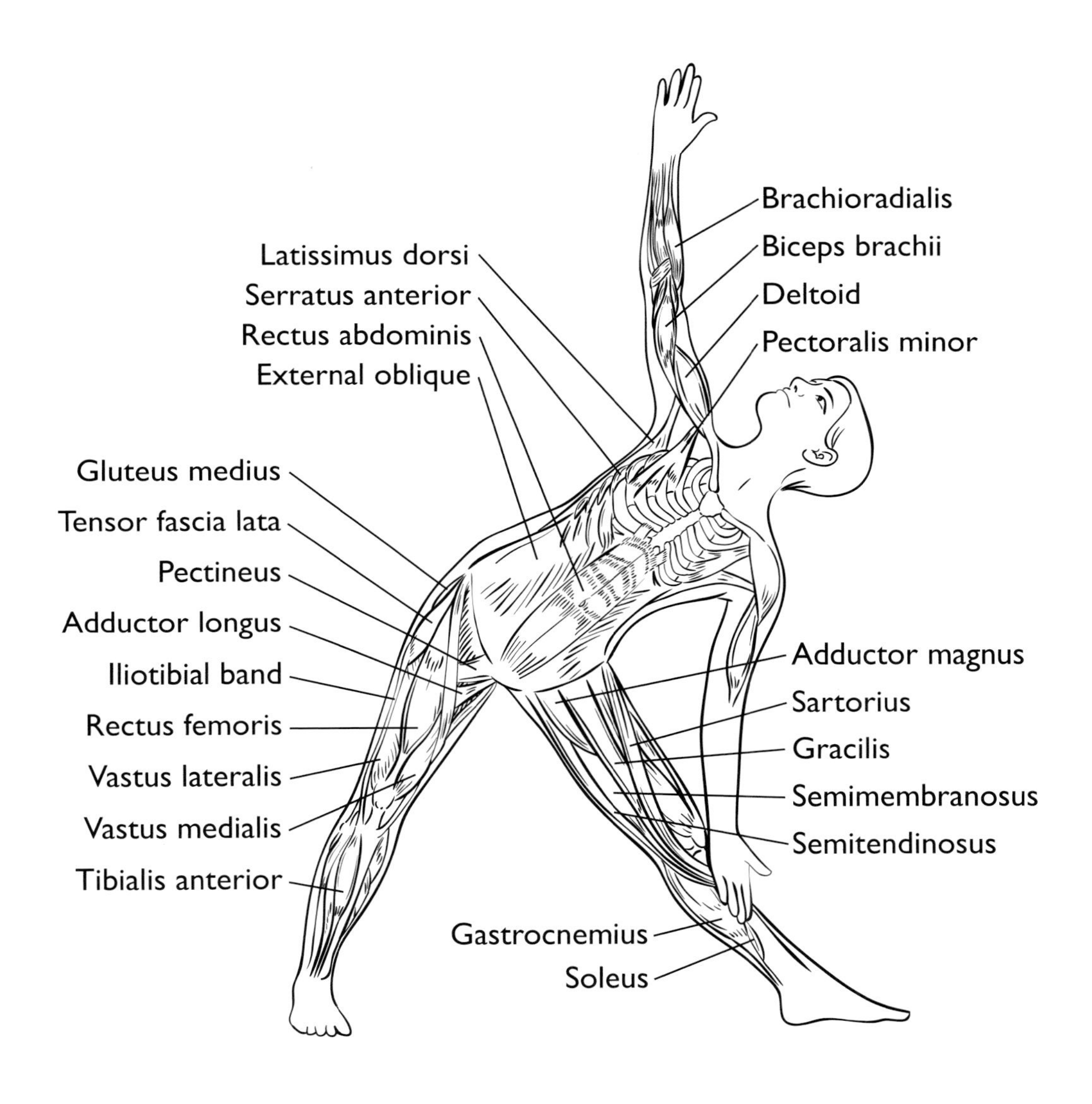

trikonasana

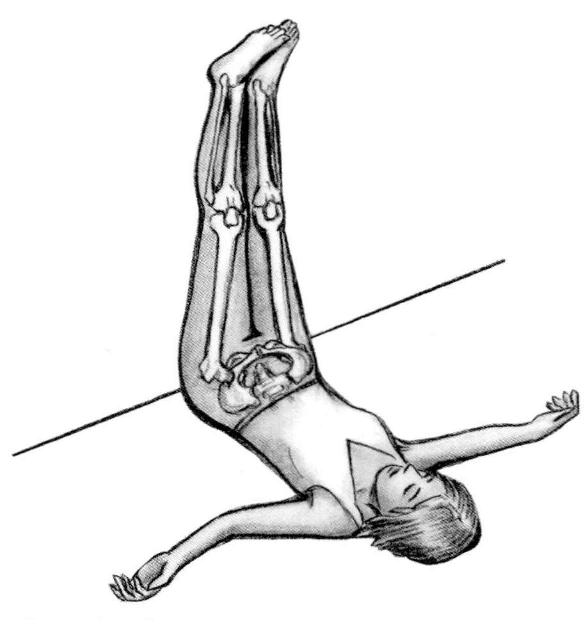

legs up the wall

Opening Relaxation: Legs Up the Wall

Come into the pose. The buttocks should be close enough to the wall so your pelvis is steady on the floor. The sacrum connects to the ground and the spine is neutral. The arms are at the sides of the body, as in Savasana.

Without bending the legs, imagine softening around the heads of the femurs in the hip sockets. Imagine gravity gently drawing the thigh bones down so that they settle comfortably into the hip sockets.

Relax and breathe for a couple of minutes.

Legs Up the Wall with Hip Release

Keeping the legs up the wall, place one ankle on top of the other. With no pelvic movement or shifting whatsoever, slowly allow the top ankle to slide down the extended leg until it stops on its own.

Breathe in place for a few minutes, focusing the attention on softening in the pelvis and hip socket; particularly of the bent leg. Observe all the sensations and any subtle (or not so subtle!) releases and changes.

Trikonasana

(Triangle Pose)

Consider your Anatomy: There are dozens of ways of moving into Trikonasana, or Triangle Pose, and to do it safely and in way that builds functional movement your focus will be at your hips -- the pelvis moving on the heads of the femurs in the most optimum way. Your knees, sacrum, sacro-iliac joints, spine, scapulae and neck will be stronger, more at ease.

Move into Trikonasana (both sides) and experience the pose. What do you feel? Where is there a feeling of being open? Is there tension or discomfort? Where? Are you struggling? How? Where is there a feeling of freedom?

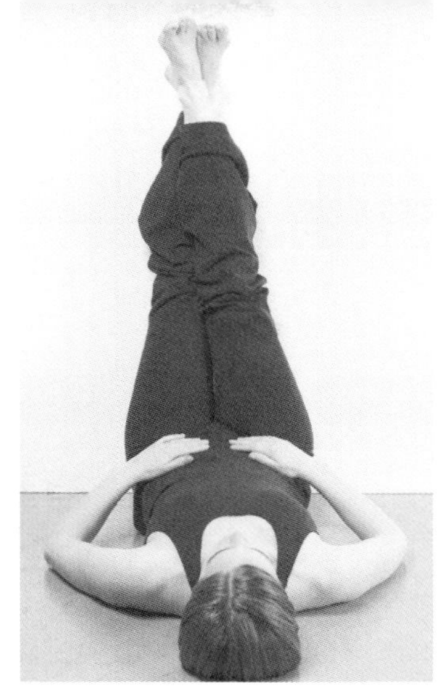

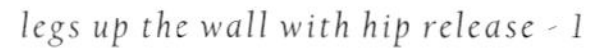

legs up the wall with hip release - 1

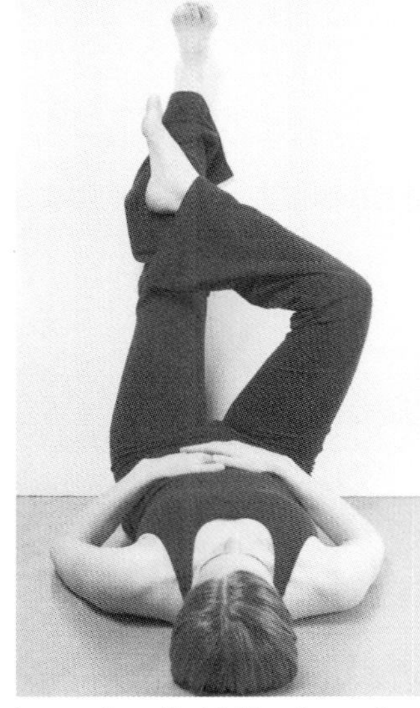

legs up the wall with hip release - 2

Slowly extend the bent leg and relax once again with both legs up the wall. Pause and observe the sensations in the left and right sides.

Change sides.

Legs Up the Wall is known as one of the more relaxing poses in yoga. See if you can transfer these feelings of relaxation into your Triangle Pose.

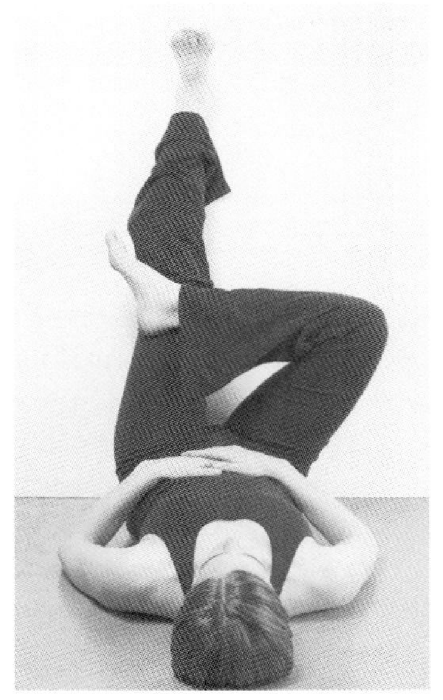

legs up the wall with hip release - 3

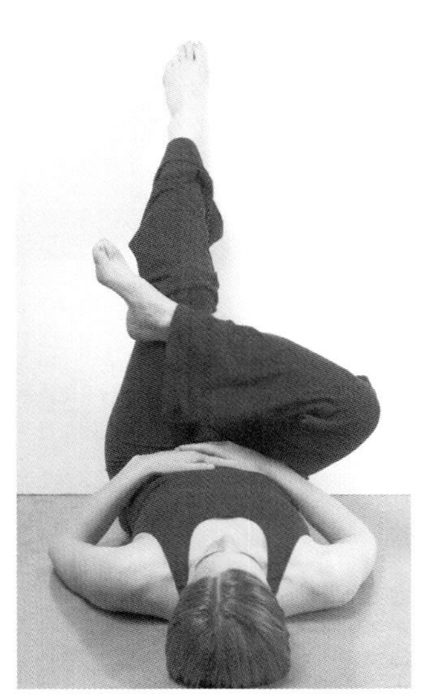

legs up the wall with hip release - 4

Pelvic Stability

Lie on your back with the knees bent and the feet planted hip width apart on the floor. The spine and pelvis are neutral.

See if you can engage the anal muscles. See if you can engage the urinary muscles. Ladies, see if you can engage the vaginal muscles. Can you distinguish between them? If one set of muscles engage, do the others necessarily engage as well? Just notice. All of these muscles gently engage in the pelvic floor lift.

Lifting the pelvic floor should not require great feats of strength. Nor does it involve any degree of pelvic tilting. It's an important but relatively gentle movement that creates pelvic stability and is useful for all poses that require pelvic stability, such as core/abdominal strengtheners and standing poses.

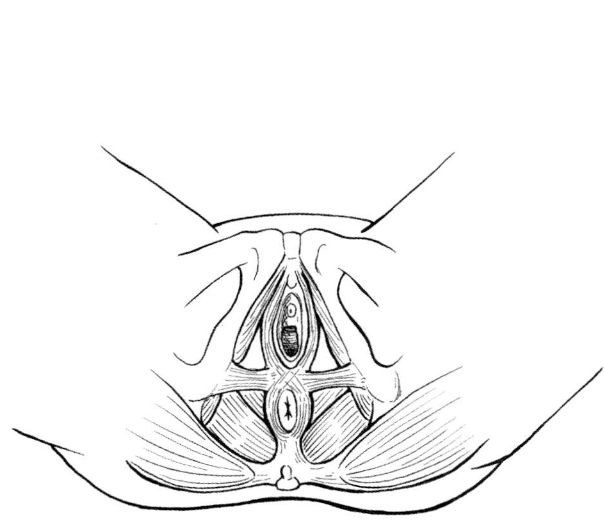

muscles of the pelvic floor - female

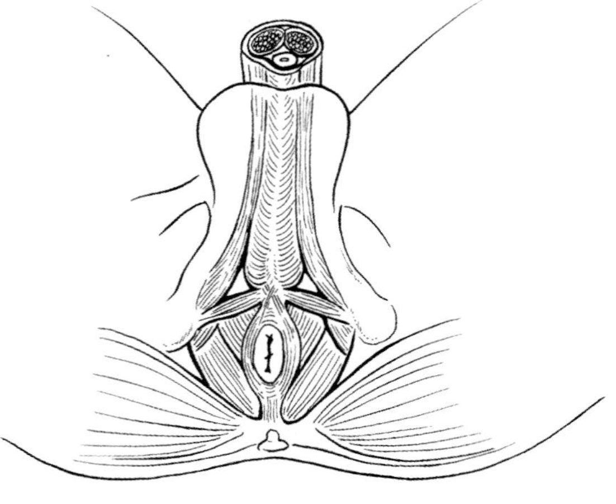

muscles of the pelvic floor - male

Keep in mind that the pelvic floor contraction needs to be balanced with a pelvic floor release. There are many men and women who have much tightness in their pelvic floor that will limit the movement and degree of support it can provide. If as you practice, you are unsure of what you are feeling or what you should be feeling, connect with a physiotherapist who specializes in the pelvic floor.

To begin: The area of the pelvic floor is both delicate and sacred. There aren't many ways to accurately describe how to engage without becoming embarrassingly graphic. Forgive my bluntness. Here we go:

Ladies: As you are laying on your back, feel with your mind's eye, the three orifices of your pelvic floor. Just in front of the anus, imagine a light, or a pool of energy collecting. As you maintain your awareness on this light or energy, you may feel this part of the pelvic floor becoming awake. Keep with your awareness. Now, gently contract all three orifices without putting out the light, without constricting your energy. You won't be contracting hard, rather it will feel gentle. Now, release, and breathe. As you continue to practice, imagine that the light is getting brighter or the energy is swelling. Then, as you release, imagine that your pelvic floor is a large water balloon which is filling. To further release the contraction, imagine the water balloon has a hole and the water drains out.

Gentlemen: This same exercise applies for you, too. You will feel the energy or light expanding and it may also feel like the center of your testicles are lifting up and into you. Again, be easy with the contraction, and fully release.

Now that the action has been described, we can practice. Try it a few times. Then, try engaging and releasing the pelvic floor in time with the breath, moving as gradually and smoothly as possible.

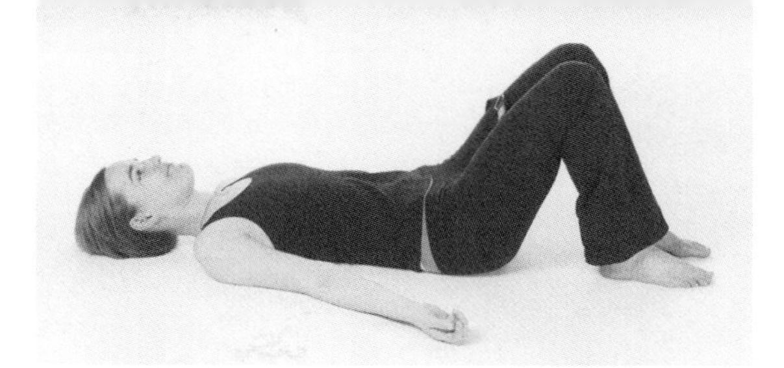

the strap

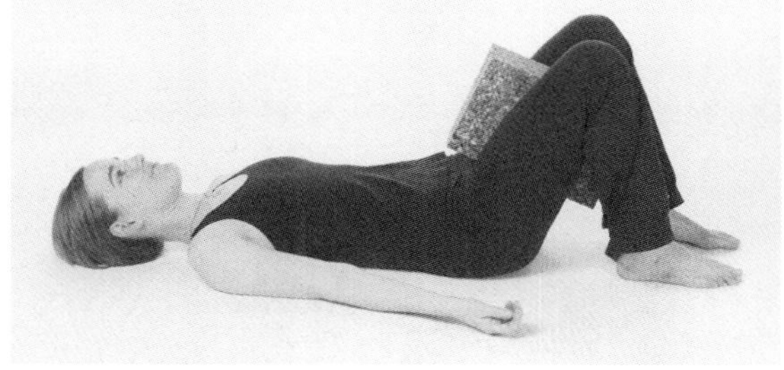

the block

The Strap

Loop and tighten a strap around both legs at the middle thigh, and return to the reclined position, as above. Place the hands on the pelvis so that the palms are flat, facing down, and the baby fingers are nestled into the hip creases. Lift one foot in the air. Can you feel the hip flexors contracting under your hand? Place the foot back on the floor. Gently press out into the strap. Notice if there was any movement or thickening of the hip flexors under the hands. There shouldn't be! The hip flexors should not be activated with this moment. Continue to gently press into the strap and release, keeping the pelvis quiet. Repeat several times.

The Block

Remove the strap and place a block in between the thighs, so that the bottom of the block is slightly above the pubic bone. Place the hands on the pelvis so that the palms are flat, facing down, and the baby fingers are nestled into the hip creases. Gently press into the block. Again, there should not be any movement of the hip flexors. Continue to gently press into the block and release, keeping the pelvis quiet. Repeat several times.

Trikonasana

(both sides)

Roll Out Hips with Tennis Ball

Stand perpendicular to the wall and place the ball between the hip and the wall. Apply pressure and observe what you feel. If you discover places that feel particularly tight, pause in place and breathe into the tightness. Move slowly left and right, up and down, exploring the whole area. Then, turn to face away from the wall, placing the ball against the back of the pelvis. Roll there.

Pause with both arms relaxed at the sides of the body and notice if there are different sensations in the left and right side.

Roll out the other side.

Pause with both arms relaxed at the sides of the body and notice the sensations.

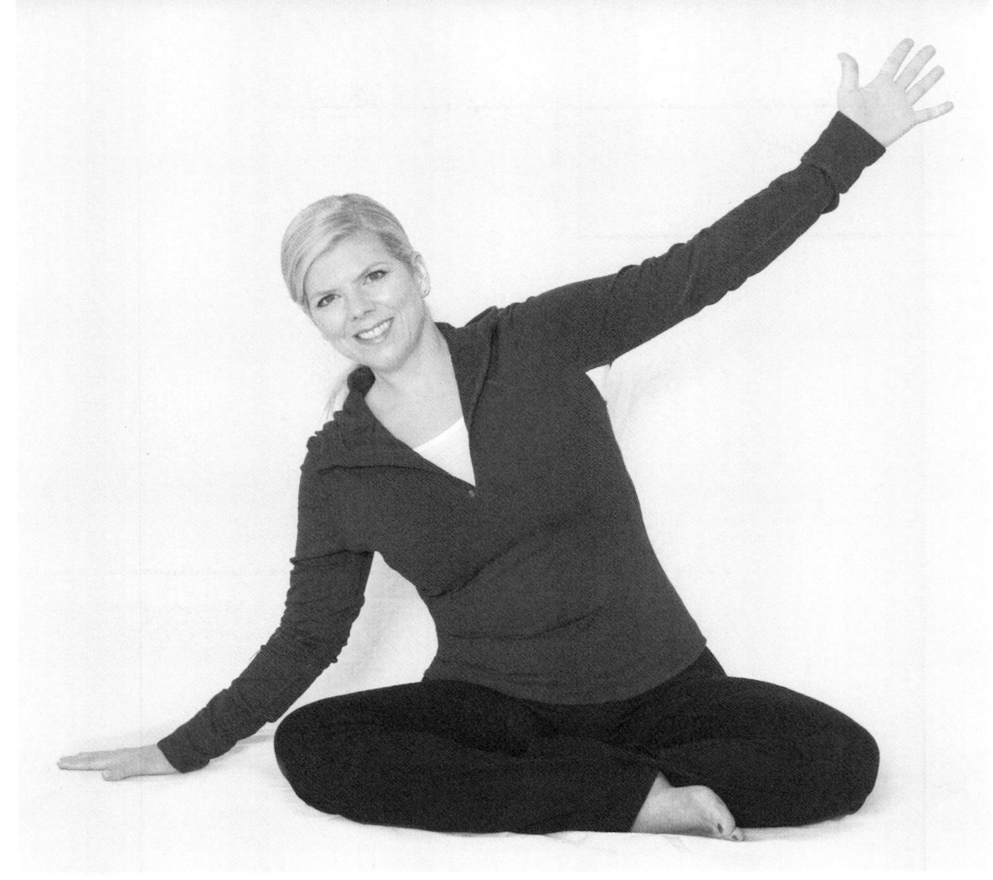

seated shoulder mobility

Trikonasana

(both sides)

Seated Shoulder Mobility

Sit comfortably and place the left hand flat on the floor about 1—1.5 feet away from the left hip, fingers facing away from the body. The shoulders are relaxed.

Keeping the left hand in position, slowly lift the straight right arm up until the arms form a diagonal line. Draw the right arm gently back into its shoulder socket. The right arm can be lowered if tension prevents this from being a comfortable position.

Slowly draw very small circles with the right arm, continuing to maintain the arm bone's connection with the shoulder socket. Repeat several times.

If it's comfortable for the neck, turn to look to the right. With the palm facing forward, slowly begin to draw the arm straight back (without moving the chest) until you reach a comfortable edge. Pause and once again draw small circles with the arm. Having circled several times, see if it's possible to take the arm back further.

Come back to centre, lower the arm and relax.

Change sides.

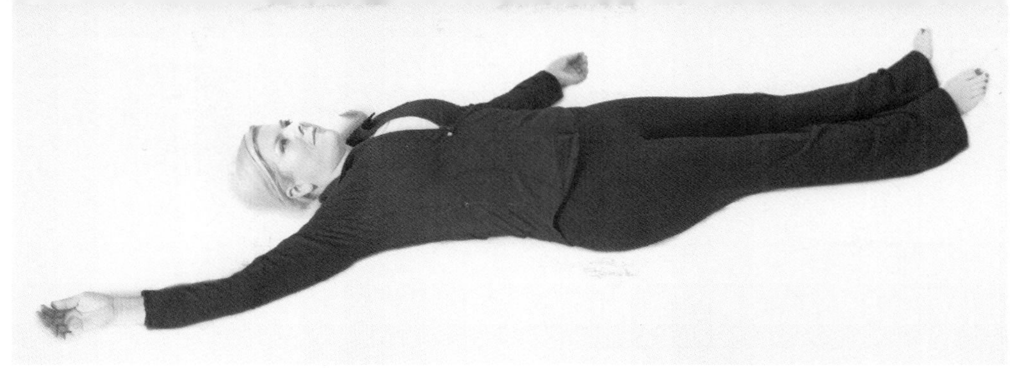

reclined crescent moon - 1

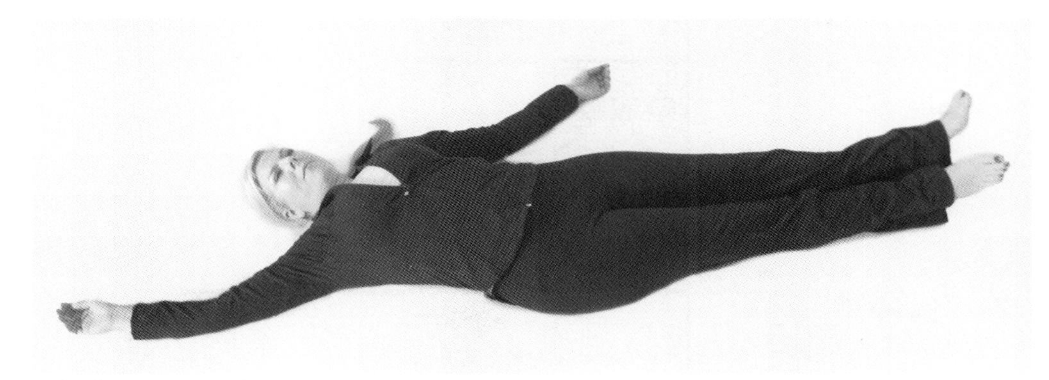

reclined crescent moon - 2

❁ *Trikonasana*

(both sides)

Reclined Crescent Moon

Lie on the mat with the legs straight out and the arms resting comfortably beside the body, palms facing up. The head is at 12 o'clock and the legs are at 6 o'clock.

Trying not to shift the pelvis, slowly move the legs to the left to 5 o'clock. Relax in place and notice if there is a stretch; most likely on the right side of the body. If there is a stretch, stay in place and breathe comfortably. If there is no stretch, slowly begin to take the right arm along the floor to shoulder height. If there is still no stretch and you are experiencing no pain, the right arm can slowly be brought up alongside the right ear on the floor, or the legs can move a little further to the left. Relax in the pose. As you inhale, imagine breathing into the place where the stretch occurs.

Come back to the original position with the head at 12 o'clock, the legs at 6 o'clock and the arms resting comfortably beside the body. Compare the sensations left to right.

Change sides.

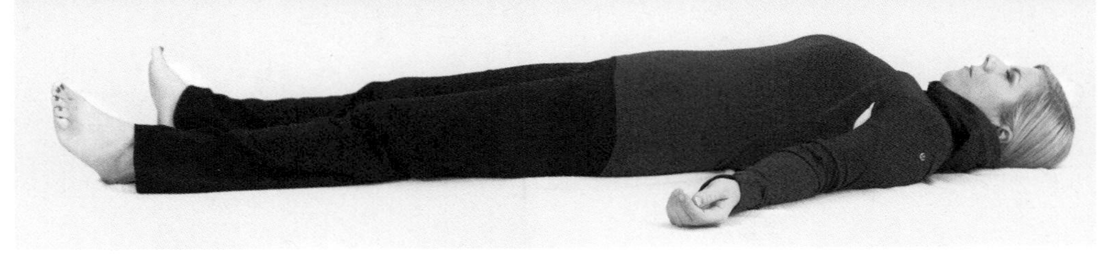

savasana

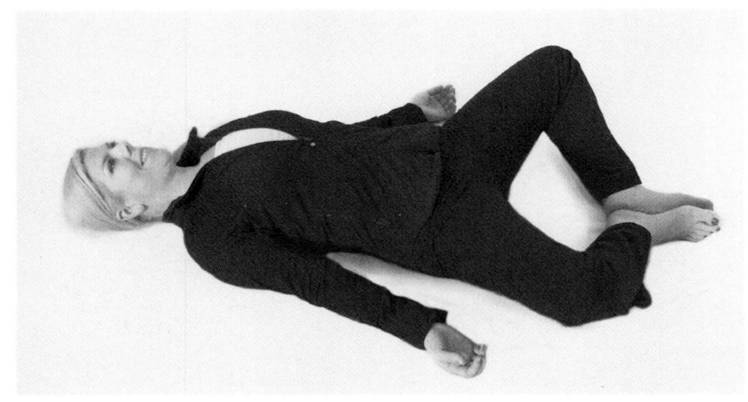

reclined bound angle

Trikonasana

(both sides)

Reclined Bound Angle

Lie on your back with the knees bent and feet planted on the ground. Slowly bring the soles of the feet together as the knees lower out to the sides. The spine should be neutral. Relax the legs and hips completely and observe the sensations.

Some people may require some support in this posture in order to feel safe and have the ability to let go. If necessary, place folded blankets or bolsters under each thigh, so that both knees are equidistant to the ground. Elevate and support the legs until a state of total relaxation can occur in the pose. You can also place a blanket under the head and neck.

Trikonasana

(both sides)

Savasana

In this Savasana, quietly focus on your breath, and become aware of your hands and feet. Be aware of the space between your eyebrows, and breathe there. Then feel your throat and neck and breathe there. Then move to your sternum and breathe there. Move to the base of the sternum and breathe there. Move to the spot 1-2" below your navel, and breathe there. Then move to your pelvic floor and breathe there. Next feel the whole centerline breathing. Let it expand outward.

Questions to consider:
How did my body feel in the various positions? Which did it enjoy, if so why? If not, why not? Am I able to differentiate between the feelings on opposites sides of my body? How does it feel to slow down and focus inward? What differences, subtle or obvious, can I feel in the pose from the first to the last instance? Do I think that I have a better awareness of the movement required to access this pose safely and effectively in my practice? Which exercise had the greatest impact, and why?

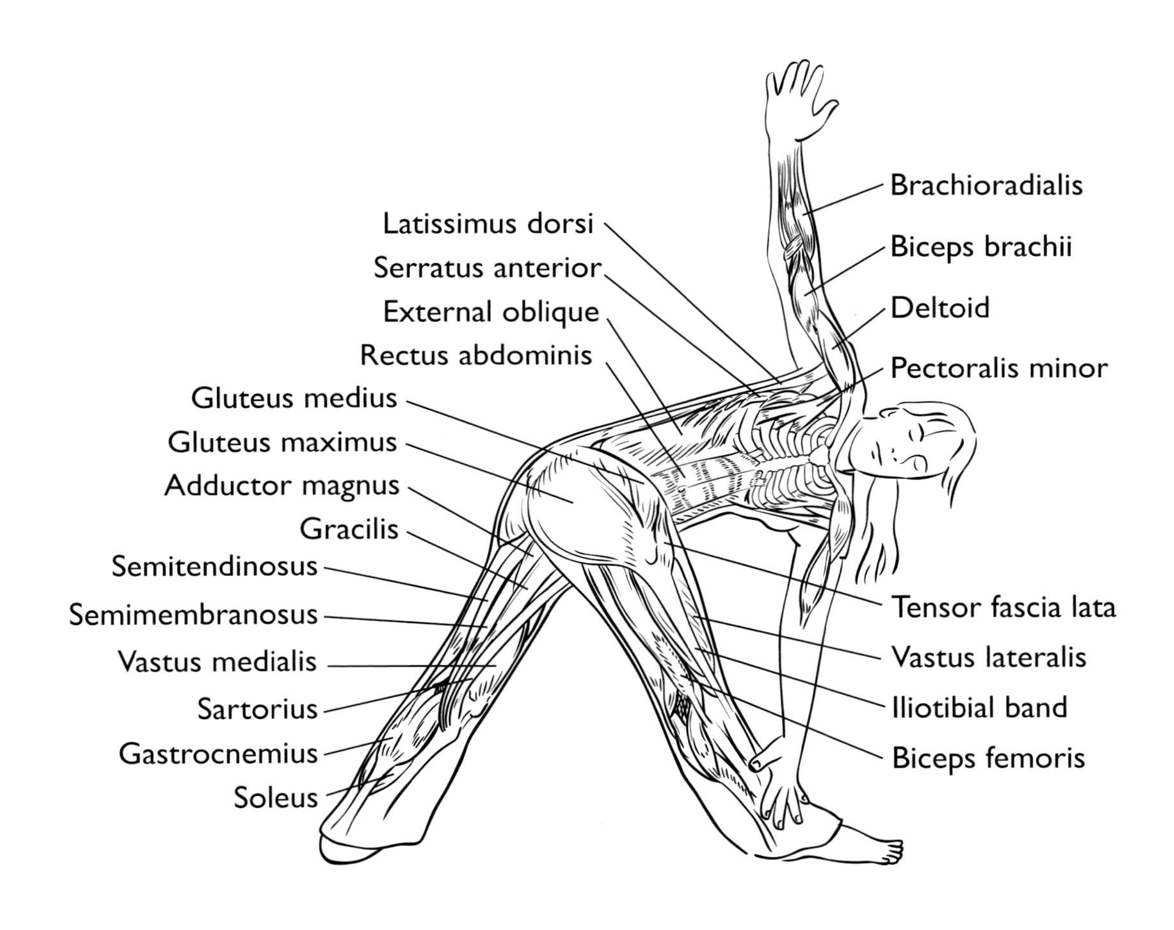

parivritta trikonasana

Parivritta Trikonasana

(Revolved Triangle)

Consider your Anatomy: Parivritta Trikonasana, or Revolved Triangle, is a complex asana in that it asks for balance, spinal rotation, and, in the full expression of the pose, the eyes gazing to the ceiling. Talk about shifting perception! The key features for safely moving into this pose include:

- good mobility and good stability of the pelvis;
- grounding through the feet for smooth motion;
- rotation of a neutral spine;
- a soft placement of the arms.

To get full access to your spinal rotators, try not to leverage too much from your arms. Whether you have placed your front hand on the floor, your ankle, shin, thigh, on a chair or wall, feel it touching whatever it is touching and "feel through" the arm. This will help to prevent gripping and overleveraging. Add the neck rotation if your collar bones are easily broad, you are feeling light, your shoulders aren't hunched and you have a steady and balanced rotation through the rest of the spine.

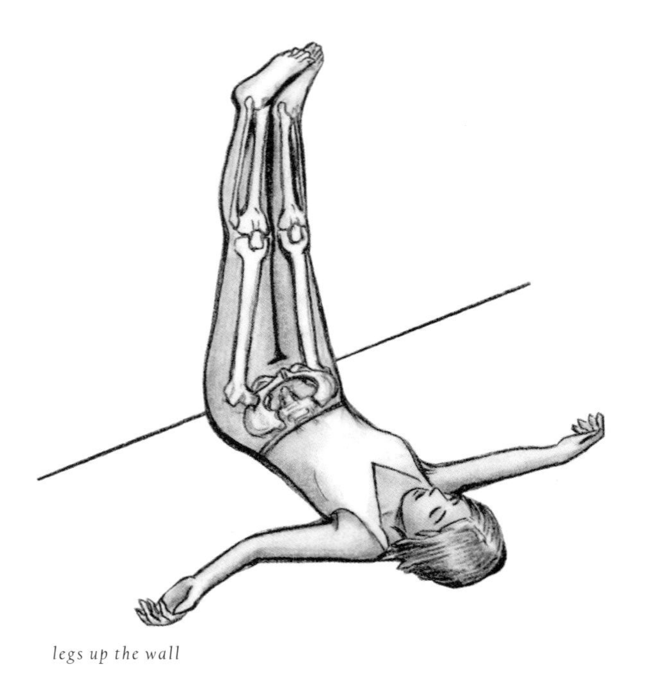

legs up the wall

To help prevent overleveraging, "feel through" the arms.

Move into Parivritta Trikonasana (both sides) and experience the pose. What do you feel? Where is there openness and freedom? Is there tension or discomfort? Where? Are you struggling? How? Where is your breath?

Opening Relaxation: Legs Up the Wall

1. Come into the pose. The position of the buttocks enables a comfortable Legs Up the Wall position, without the hips lifting. The back of your pelvis will feel like it is connecting to the ground and the spine is neutral. The arms are at the sides of the body, as in Savasana. If there is a jamming sensation or strain around or near the sacrum or sacroiliac joints, ease back.

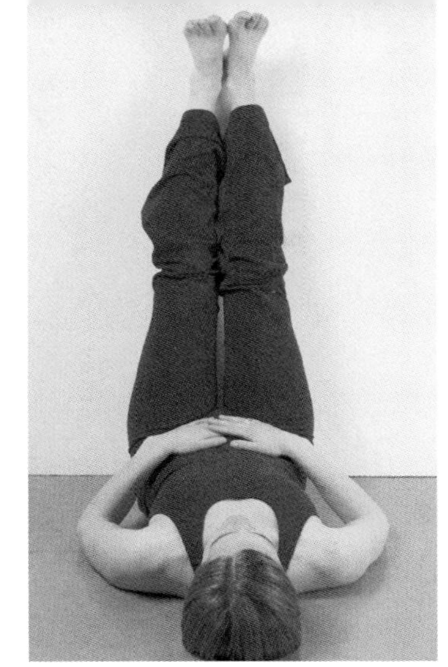

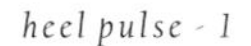

heel pulse - 1

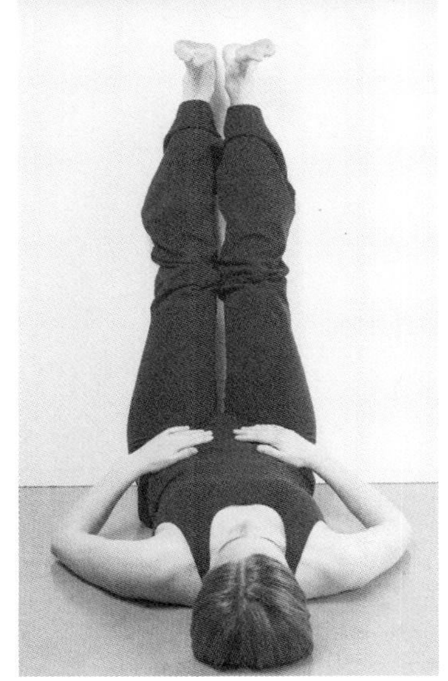

heel pulse - 2

2. Without bending the legs, imagine softening around the heads of the femurs in the hip sockets. Imagine your pelvis is like clay and your legs are like dowling and the dowling is sinking into the clay.

3. Relax and breathe for several minutes.

Heel Pulse

1. Keeping the legs up the wall, reach up with the heels, pressing them to the ceiling, coming into dorsal flexion, then relax. Keep the toes as easy as possible.

2. Repeat five to ten times, moving gently with the breath.

Parivritta Trikonasana

(both sides)

Shoulder and Torso Movements

1. Lie on the mat in a fetal position on the left side.

2. Support the head with a folded blanket so the neck is in a neutral position. Knees are bent with one knee on top of the other.

3. Extend the arms out in front of the body at shoulder height, resting on the floor. The arms are straight and the bottom (left) palm faces the sky. The top (right) palm rests face down on the left hand.

Arm Reaches:

4. Exhale as you slowly reach the top hand beyond the bottom hand. The movement is probably not more than a few inches.

5. Inhale as you draw the top hand back to its starting position.

6. Repeat several times. While your hand and arm are what you see moving, the movement is initiating at your shoulder blades.

7. Legs stay stable and the ribs are quiet. If movement occurs in either area, make the arm reaches smaller until movement is isolated to the shoulder blade and arm.

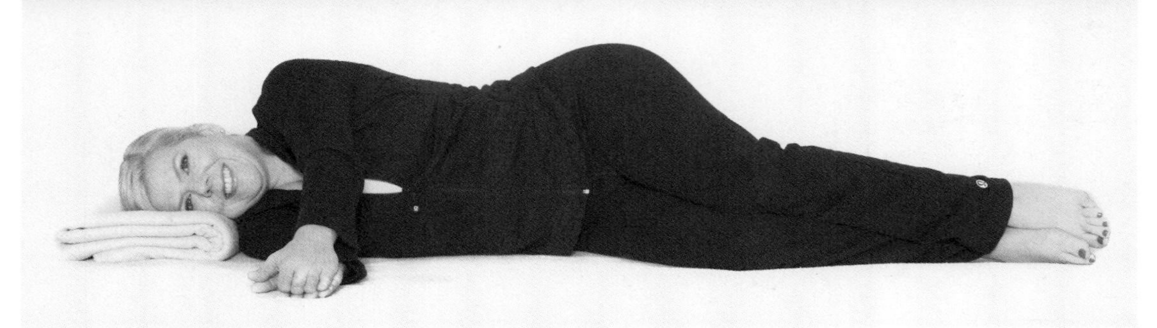

shoulder and torso movements - arm reaches

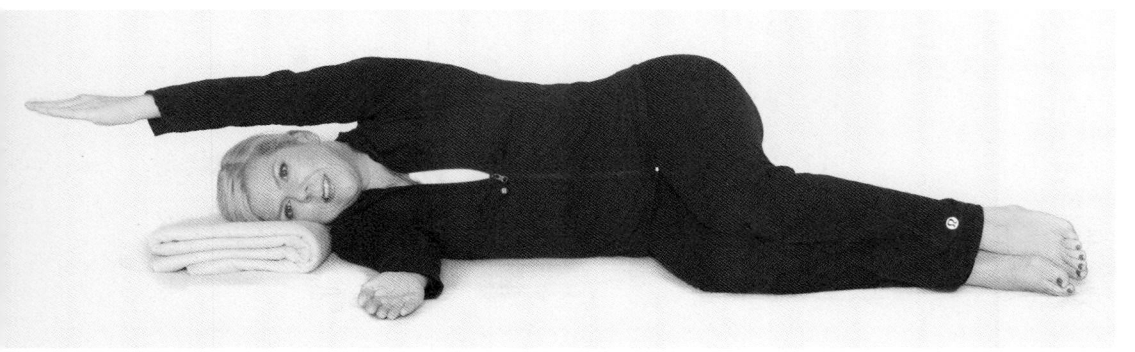

shoulder and torso movements - arm arcs

Arm Arcs:

8. Return to the original position with one arm on top of the other on the floor at shoulder height.

9. Lift the top arm shoulder height above the bottom arm that remains on the floor.

10. Slowly begin to arc the top arm until it comes alongside the ear. Repeat several times.

Note:
If clicking, pain, general wonkiness or backbending occur, make the arcs smaller until a pain-free, click-free, non-backbending movement can occur. It might be necessary to elevate the top arm higher than shoulder height above the floor, or to slightly bend the elbow to accomplish this.

Think of easily breathing from the inside of your ribs using your breath as a guide to sustain the position of your ribs so they don't flair forward.

Twist:

11. Return to the original position with one arm on top of the other on the floor at shoulder height.

12. Keeping the top arm bone drawn into its shoulder socket, slowly begin to lift this arm straight up toward the sky.

13. When the arm is at the sky, begin to twist. Initiate the twist from the spine, allowing the arm to follow. Think of the chest opening, without back bending. Continue to move the arm only as far as the spine rotates. If the spine stops rotating, stop moving the arm.

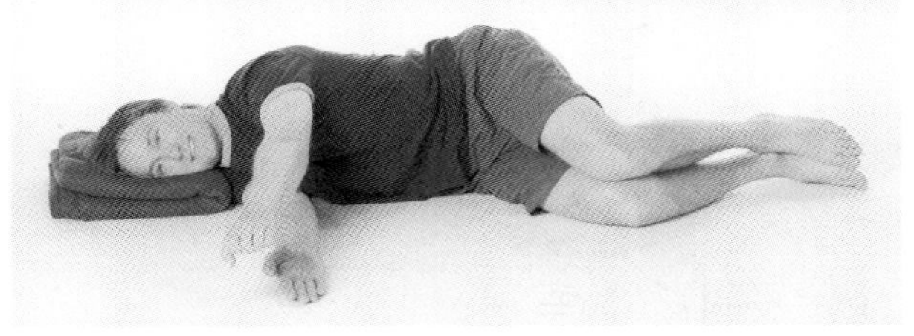

shoulder and torso movements - twist - 1

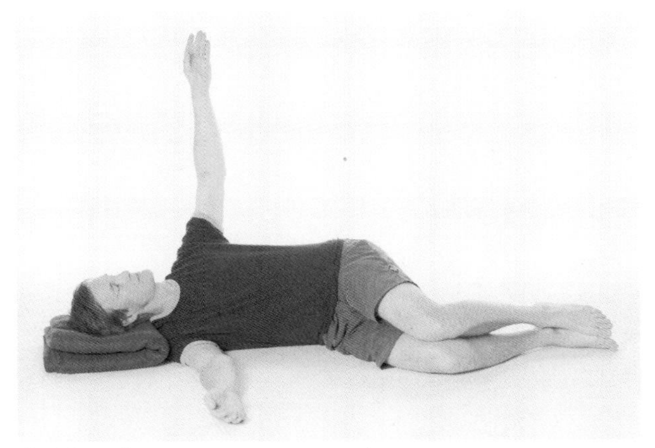

shoulder and torso movements - twist - 2

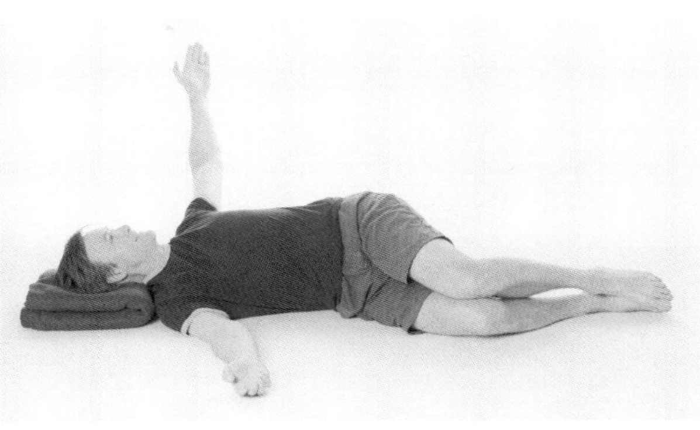

shoulder and torso movements - twist - 3

14. You can experiment with either breathing in place and experiencing the sensations, or repeating the movement several times from the beginning.

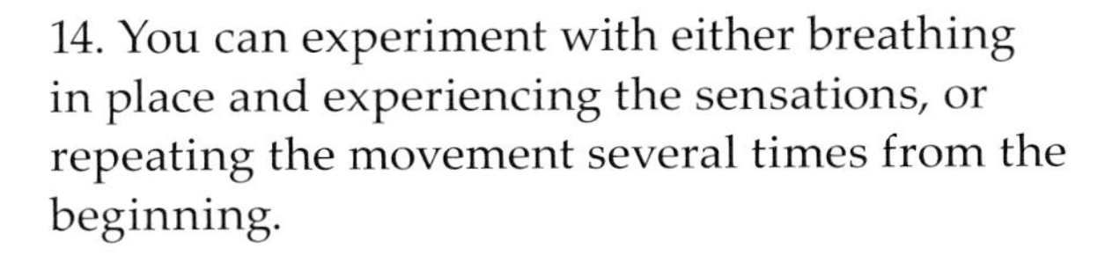

Note:

- The legs should not move. The top leg and hip may start to draw back as the twist deepens. The ideal range of motion in the spine occurs within a movement-free range of motion in the pelvis and legs. If you have SI joint issues only move through the range of motion that is pain-free and easy.

- The twisting movement is initiated from the spine. Ensure that the shoulder or arm don't lead the motion.

- The top arm should always remain in line with the shoulder, and not lead the twisting movement or be allowed to dangle in space.

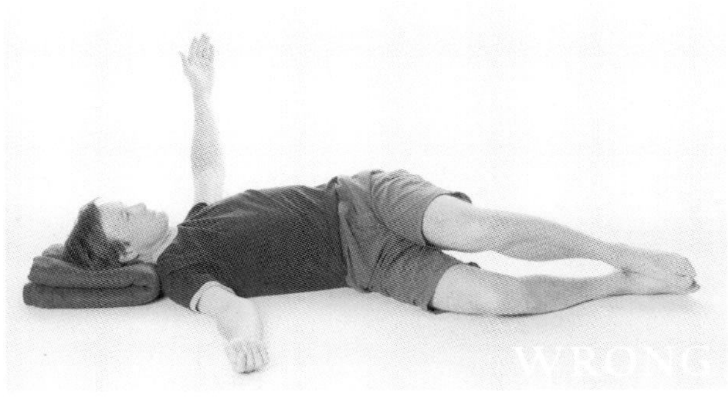

wrong - knees are lifting

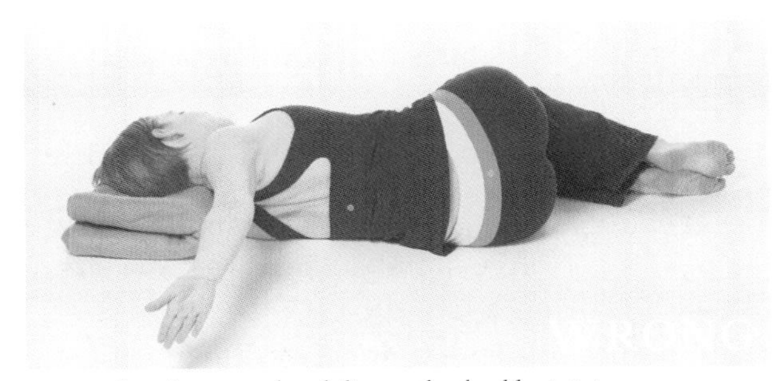

wrong - there is too much mobility at the shoulder joint

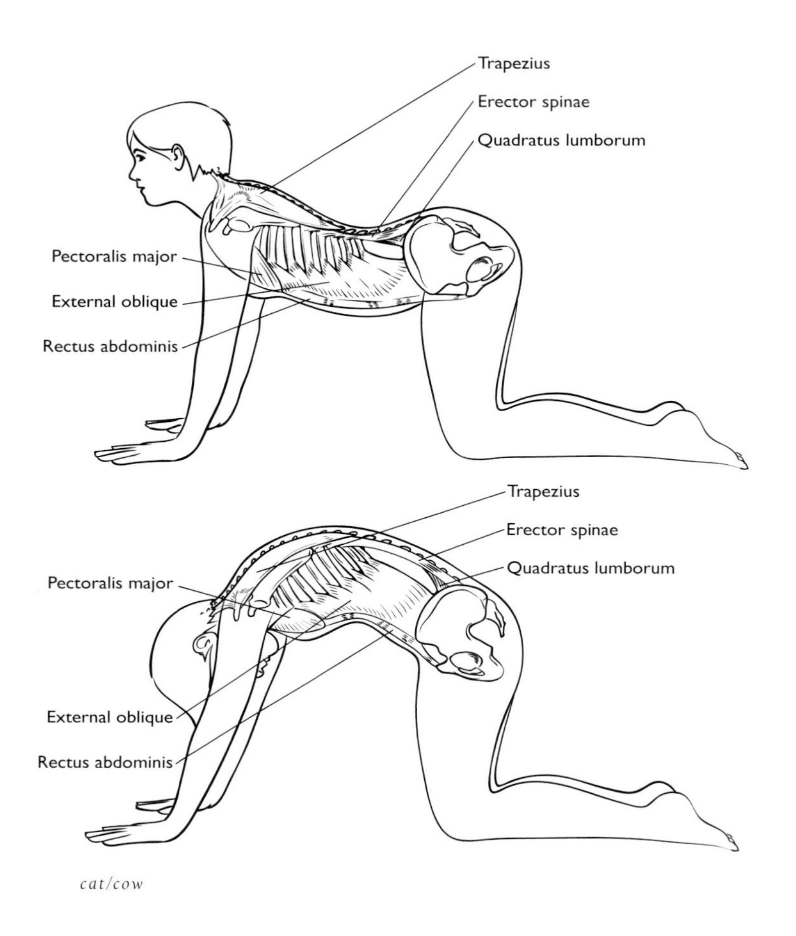

cat/cow

Parivritta Trikonasana

(both sides)

Cat/Cow

1. Come into Table pose on the hands and knees, with the wrists beneath the shoulders and the knees beneath the hips.

2. Exhale as you slowly start to lower the tailbone and head, arching upward like an angry cat. Press up between the shoulder blades coming into the apex of the pose.

3. Inhale as you slowly move the spine in the opposite direction, tilting the tailbone towards the sky, lengthing through the spine, and gently lifting the gaze, as you come into spinal extension.

Note: This series of movements should never create sensations of compression or pain in or along the spine. If this occurs, encourage the intention of lengthening and creating space and/ or make the movement smaller.

Consider: The intention behind the movement can create different experiences in this simple flow. Try several rounds leading the movement with the head and neck. Try several more rounds leading the movement with the tailbone. Imagine breathing between your shoulder blades and up along your spine as you move. Feel the flow of your breath as if it is water moving fluidly.

Side Stretch Variations from Table

1. Come into Table pose, as directed in the previous exercise.

2. Keeping the pelvis and legs in place, move the hands and shoulders 45 degrees to the right, so that the wrists are directly beneath the shoulders and fingers point straight out to the side.

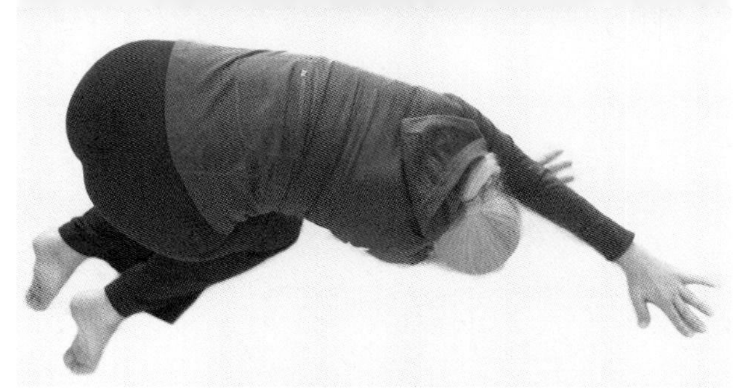

side stretch variations from table - 1

side stretch variations from table - 2

side stretch variations from table - modification

side stretch variations from table - modification

3. Lower the right forearm down on a diagonal.

4. Lower the forehead onto this forearm. You may need to move the forearm slightly further away from the body for it to provide a comfortable resting place for the head.

5. Keeping the pelvis above the knees (don't drop back into Child Pose!), slowly start to extend the left arm straight out to the right side.

6. The arm will probably come alongside the left ear. Place the left palm flat on the ground and observe the sensations along the left side of the body.

7. Different types of opening can occur in this position by pressing out gently in the following ways: Try pressing gently out with the left hip. Pause in place and observe the sensations. Then try pressing out with the left waist, rib cage and underarm. Pause in place and observe the sensations caused by each separate area of focus.

8. Return to Table or Child Pose and relax for several breaths.

Change sides.

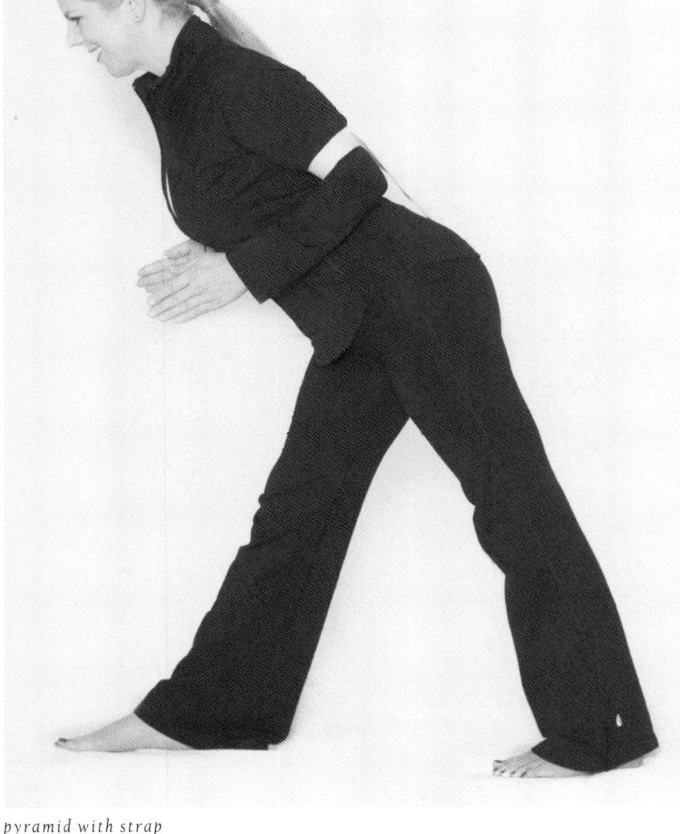

pyramid with strap

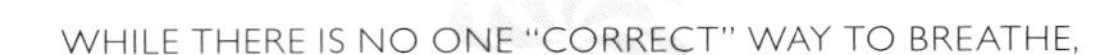

WHILE THERE IS NO ONE "CORRECT" WAY TO BREATHE,

THERE ARE MORE AND LESS EFFECTIVE WAYS OF BREATHING.

—Donna Farhi

Parivritta Trikonasana

(both sides)

Pyramid with Strap

1. Stay standing and loop a strap around the arms just above the elbows. Tighten the strap enough so that the elbows are drawn into the sides of the body and a sense of openness occurs in the chest. Allow your palms to face in.

2. Stand with the feet hip width apart and take a step back with the left foot, ensuring that the hips remain equidistant to the floor and the wall in front of you.

3. Pressing into the back heel and grounding into the four corners of the front foot, slowly begin to hinge forward from the hip crease.

4. The spine remains neutral throughout.

5. Pause in place when you start to feel a stretch, taking care that the left hip has not pulled back.

6. Observe the sensations as you take several breaths in place.

7. Slowly release the pose and change sides.

8. Having completed the second side, carefully remove the strap and stand in Mountain. Observe the sensations in the body. Is there a greater sense of openness in the chest than before? Is it easier to breathe? Do the shoulders sit differently?

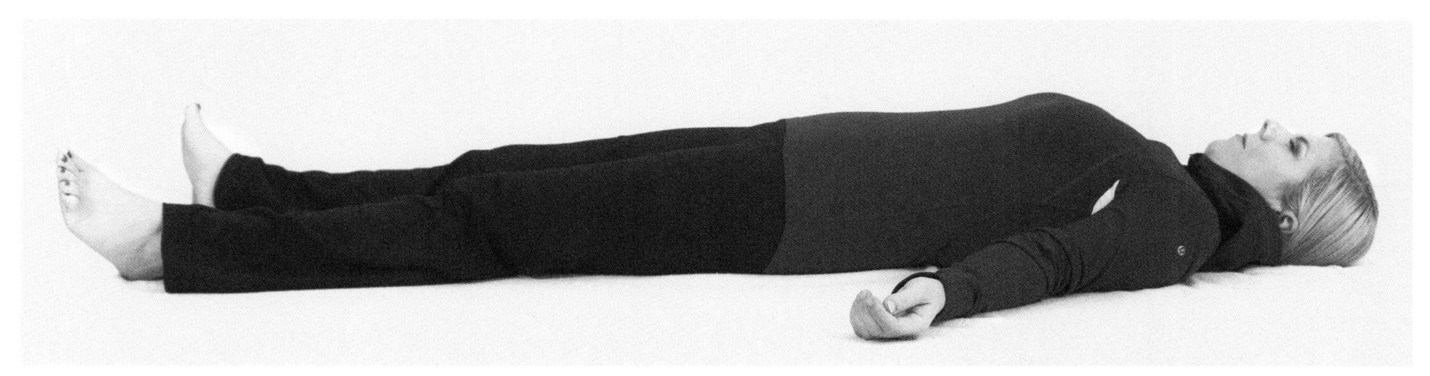

savasana

֍ *Parivritta Trikonasana*

(both sides)

Savasana

On your back, bring your attention to your breath. Then, place your hands on your lower belly, between your navel and pubic bone. Become aware of your breath in this area, Then, feel the breath slightly laterally at the edges of where the pelvis meets the belly. After several breaths, become aware of how the breath moves directly behind the naval and lower back. Now bring your attention to all sides of your lower belly – front, sides and back. Can you feel the entire circumference breathing? Let this technique go, and be still – feel and be aware.

Questions to consider:
How did my body feel in the various positions? Which did it enjoy, and if so why? If not, why not? Could I differentiate the spinal motion and the shoulder motion when I twisted? Was I able to feel a connection between the myofascia of the chest releasing and shoulder mobility? How did Parivritta Trikonasana change as I went through the practice? Am I able to differentiate between the feelings on opposites sides of my body? How does it feel to slow down and focus inward? What differences, subtle or obvious, can I feel in the pose from the first to the last instance? Do I think that I have a better awareness of the movement required to access this pose safely and effectively in my practice? Which exercise had the greatest impact, and why?

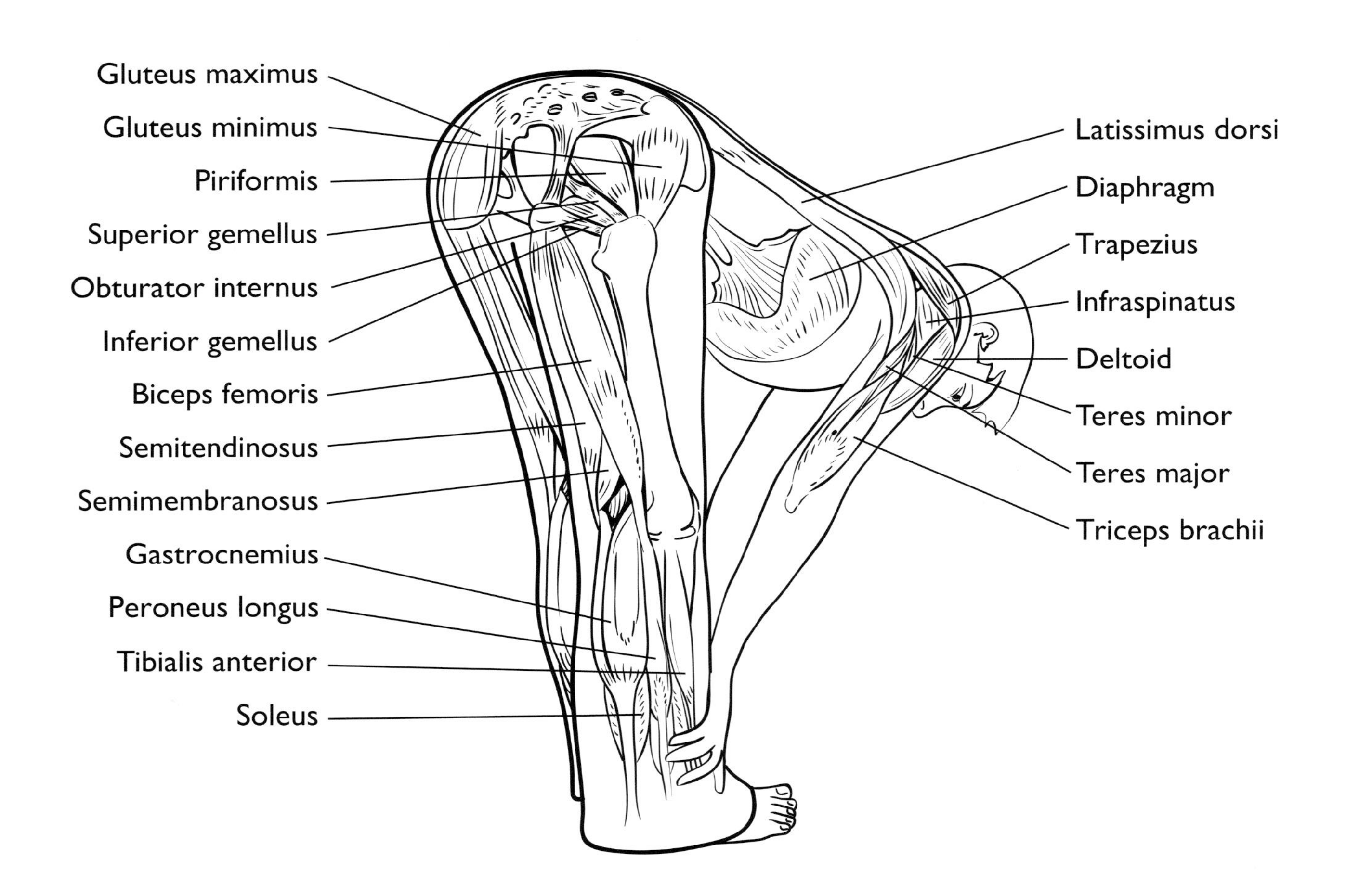
Gluteus maximus
Gluteus minimus
Piriformis
Superior gemellus
Obturator internus
Inferior gemellus
Biceps femoris
Semitendinosus
Semimembranosus
Gastrocnemius
Peroneus longus
Tibialis anterior
Soleus
Latissimus dorsi
Diaphragm
Trapezius
Infraspinatus
Deltoid
Teres minor
Teres major
Triceps brachii

uttanasana

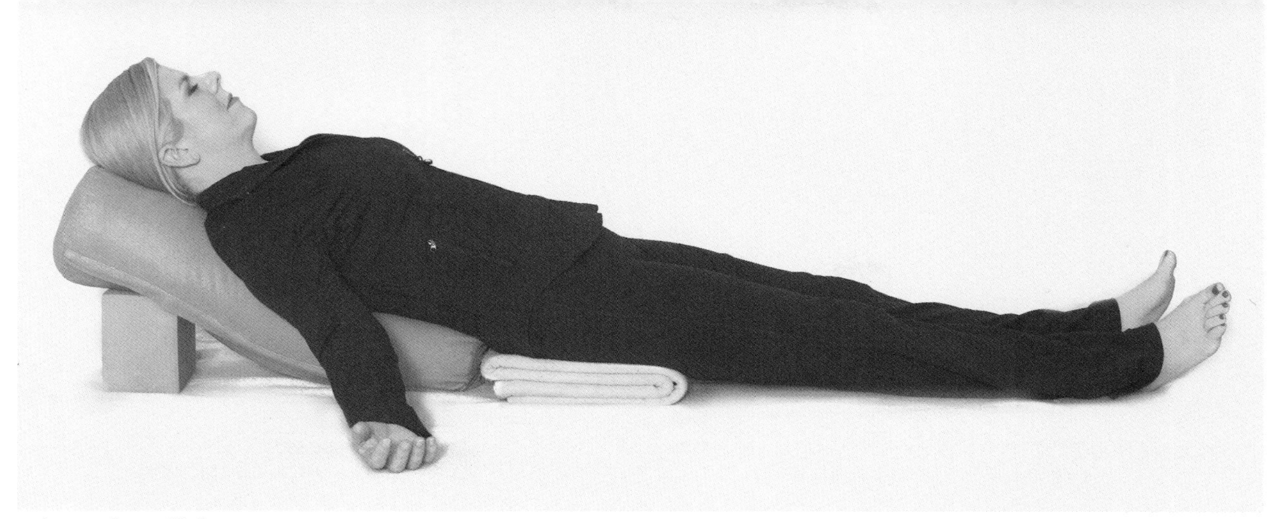

recline on elevated bolster

Uttanasana

(Standing Forward Bend)

Consider your Anatomy: Uttanasana, or Standing Forward Bend, is a terrific pose for lengthening the back line of your body. And, while we don't often consider it a pure balance posture, balance is a key feature if the back line – plantar fascia, gastrocnemius, hamstrings, gluteal muscles, and erector spinae are all going to release and allow for deeper experience of the pose. Remember that as you move forward this back line of muscles will be eccentrically contracting in order to control your forward descent. Your ability to connect to your core – particularly how your pelvic stability engages with your feet – will help you move safely and deeply.

Move into Uttanasana and experience the pose. Where do you feel movement and freedom? Is there tension or discomfort? Where? Are you struggling? How?

Opening Relaxation: Recline on Elevated Bolster

1. Place a bolster parallel with the mat, toward the top of the mat.

2. Elevate the top end of the bolster with a block.

3. Place a folded blanket on the mat at the bottom end of the bolster.

4. Sit on the blanket with the lower back against the bolster and legs extended on the mat.

5. Recline onto the bolster.

6. If necessary, place another folded blanket under the head or under the forearms.

7. Relax, breathe easy and allow the body to settle for several minutes.

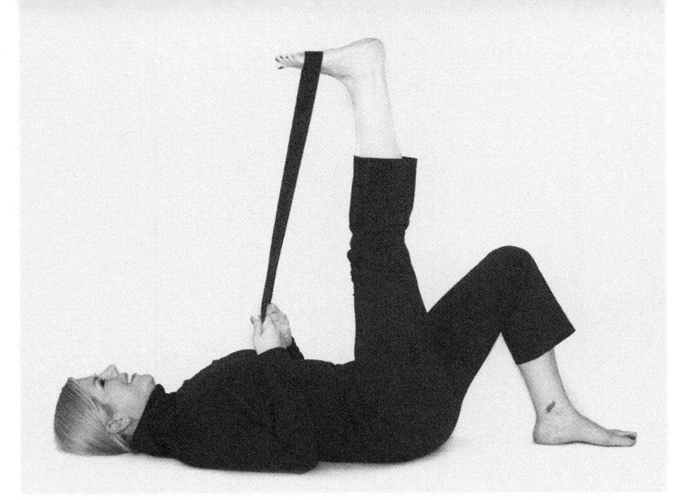

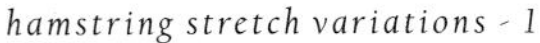

hamstring stretch variations - 1

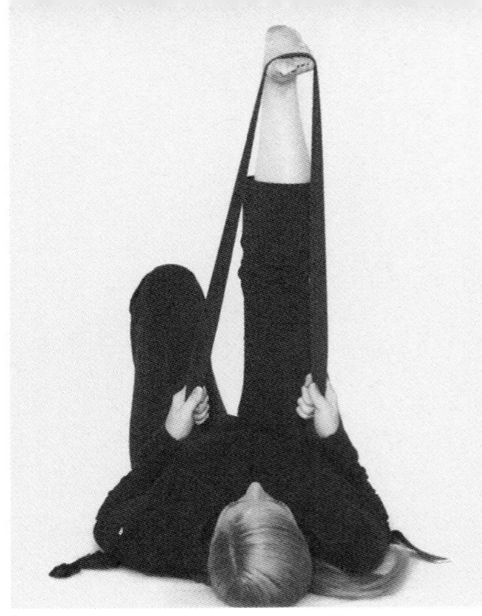

hamstring stretch variations - 2

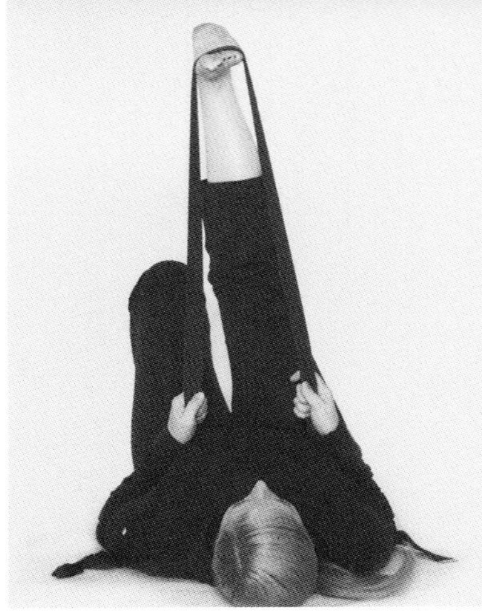

hamstring stretch variations - 3

Roll out the Feet with Tennis Ball

1. Stand up and place a tennis ball under one foot.

2. Roll the foot on the tennis ball and observe what you feel. If you discover places that feel particularly tight, pause in place, breathe, and smile.

3. Move slowly left and right, up and down, exploring the entire underside of the foot for a couple of minutes.

4. Pause and stand in Tadasana comparing the sensations in the feet, legs and pelvis.

5. Come into Uttanasana and compare the two sides.

6. Return to standing and roll out the other foot.

7. Pause and stand in Tadasana comparing the sensations in the feet, legs and pelvis.

8. Come into Uttanasana, comparing the two sides and noticing the sensations. Has the pose changed? How? Do you feel more connected with the ground? In standing imagine you have energetic roots and they are moving into the floor and to the core of the earth, they then rebound back into you, bringing the earth's energy to you. Feel this through your legs and pelvis.

Hamstring Stretch Variations

1. Lie on the mat with both knees bent and the feet planted hip width apart.

2. Bend the right knee toward the chest and place a strap around the ball of the right foot.

3. Slowly extend the leg straight up to the sky.

4. Pause in place and imagine the right thigh bone nestling down into the right hip socket. The sacrum is flat on the floor and the spine is neutral.

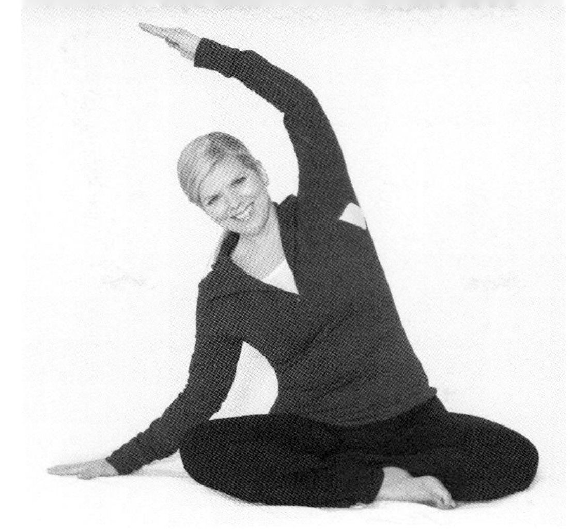

seated side stretches - 1

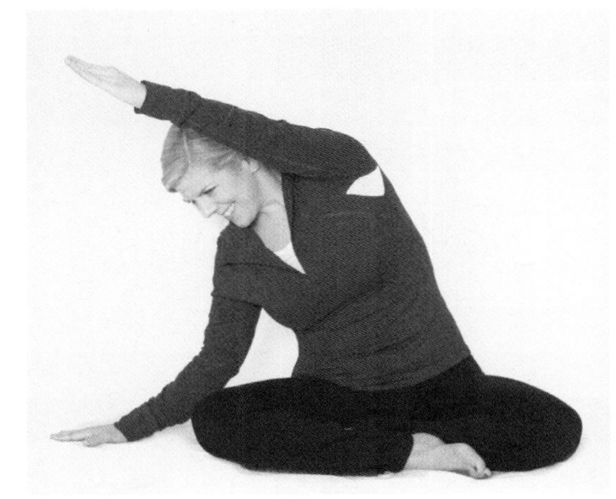

seated side stretches - 2

5. Gently reach up with the right heel, while simultaneously pressing the ball of the right foot gently into the strap.

6. Relax in place, noticing the sensations, and breathe easily for one to three minutes.

7. To enhance your awareness of subtle movement, observe the epicentre of the stretch.

8. Continuing your observation, slowly move the leg a couple of inches to the left. The pelvis should stay evenly grounded throughout.

9. Slowly come out of the pose, extend the legs on the mat, and observe the sensations from left to right.

Change sides.

Breathe and be easy, strong, supple and still.

Uttanasana

(both sides)

Seated Side Stretches

1. Sit comfortably and place the left hand flat on the floor about 1—1.5 feet away from the left hip, fingers facing away from the body. The shoulders are relaxed.

2. Keeping the left hand in position, slowly arc the straight right arm up until it comes across the right ear. The palm faces down and the right arm is active, with the arm bone drawn into its shoulder socket.

3. Ensure that the right hip/pelvis don't lift or tilt off the floor. Keep them grounded.

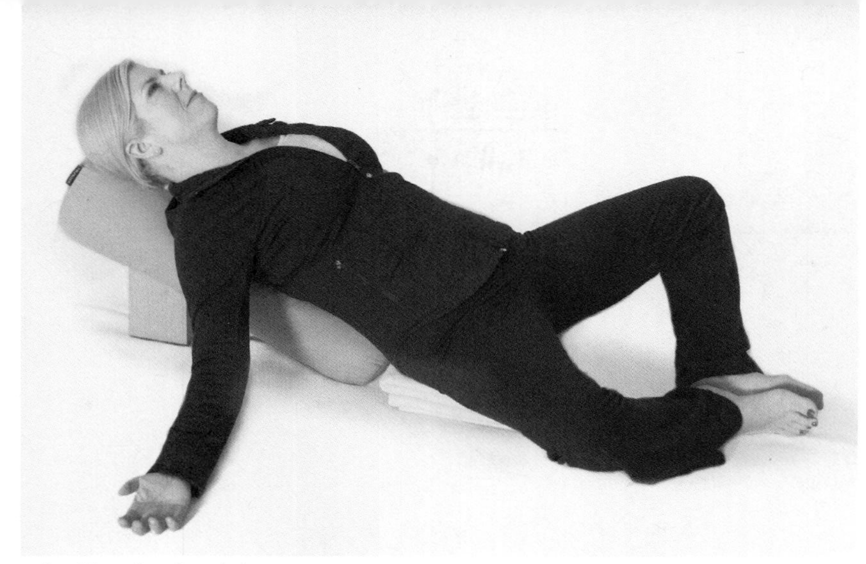

reclined bound angle on bolster

4. Observe the sensations, as you gently inhale to expand the stretch on the right side, exhaling to release.

5. Stay in this position and reach the right arm out in a diagonal line to the left. Observe the sensations, as you gently inhale to expand the stretch on the right side, exhaling to relax.

6. Come back to centre and lower the arm.

Change sides.

Uttanasana

(both sides)

Something to explore: Place a block between your legs one inch from your pubic bone. Don't squeeze hard – simply hold it. Now move into Uttanasana. What did you feel?

Reclined Bound Angle on Bolster

1. Place a bolster parallel with the mat, toward the top of the mat. Elevate the top end of the bolster with a block. Place a folded blanket on the mat at the bottom end of the bolster.

2. Sit on the blanket with the lower back against the bolster.

3. Recline onto the bolster.

4. Bend knees and place the soles of the feet together, allowing the hips to soften and the knees to drop out to the sides.

5. If necessary, place another folded blanket under the head and one bolster under each thigh. Relax, breathe easy and allow the body to settle for a couple of minutes.

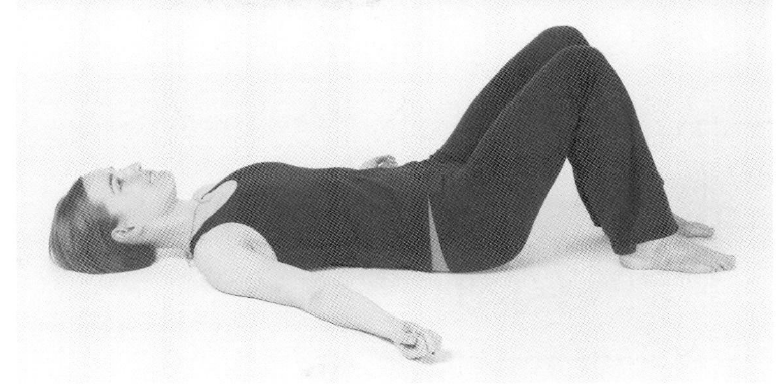

butterfly - 1

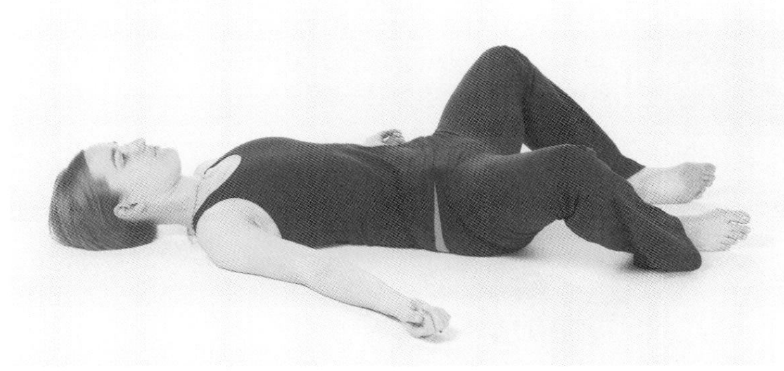

butterfly - 2

Butterfly

1. Remove the bolster and lie back with the knees bent and feet planted close together on the mat.

2. Take five full breaths to slowly lower the knees outward into Bound Angle.

3. Take 15 full breaths to slowly bring the knees back up to their original position.

4. Repeat three to five times.

5. There may be some shaking in the legs as you do this exercise which is often a myofascial release. Stick with it and you'll find over time the shaking subsiding and your hips releasing.

Consider: When you move slowly, mindfully, and gently through a yoga asana, you give the muscular and fascial (myofascia) structures of your body a chance to release. The experience is often one of "more space". When we move quickly or we force, the myofascia provides rigid resistance. Play with this and see what transpires in your practice.

THIS CALM STEADINESS OF THE SENSES IS CALLED YOGA.

THEN ONE SHOULD BECOME WATCHFUL, BECAUSE YOGA COMES AND GO.

—*Katha Upanishad*

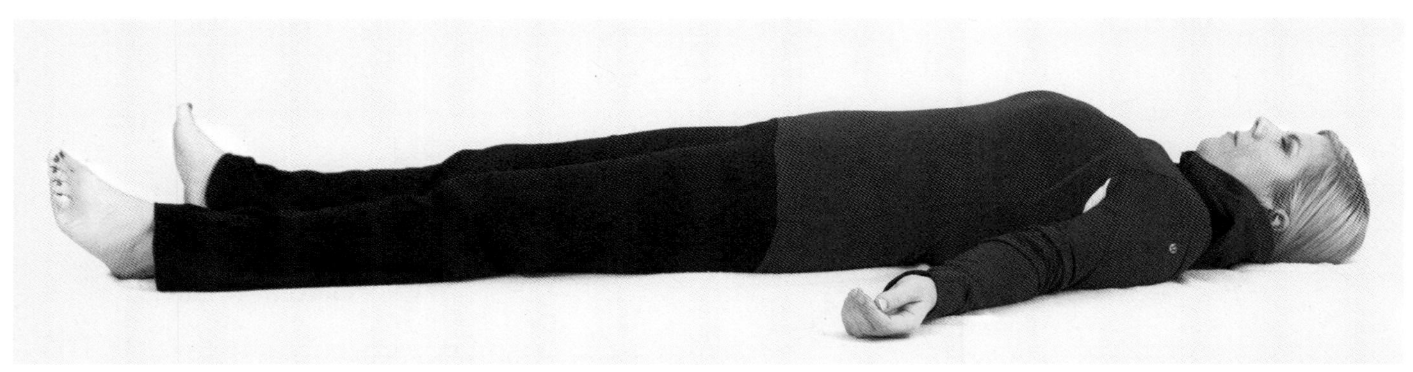

savasana

Uttanasana

(both sides)

Savasana

As you lay back, feel the front and back of your body — feel yourself touching the floor and feel the front of you opening to the sky. Feel the space between the front and the back. Watch the breath percolate in this space, however it does.

Questions to consider:
How did my feet feel during and after using the tennis ball? Was there a residual release occurring further up the leg or into the torso after using the tennis ball? How did my body feel in Standing Forward Bend following the various explorations? Which did it enjoy, if so why? If not, why not? Am I able to differentiate between the feelings on opposites sides of my body? How does it feel to slow down and focus inward? What differences, subtle or obvious, can I feel in the pose from the first to the last instance? Do I think that I have a better awareness of the movement required to access this pose safely and effectively in my practice? Which exercise had the greatest impact, and why?

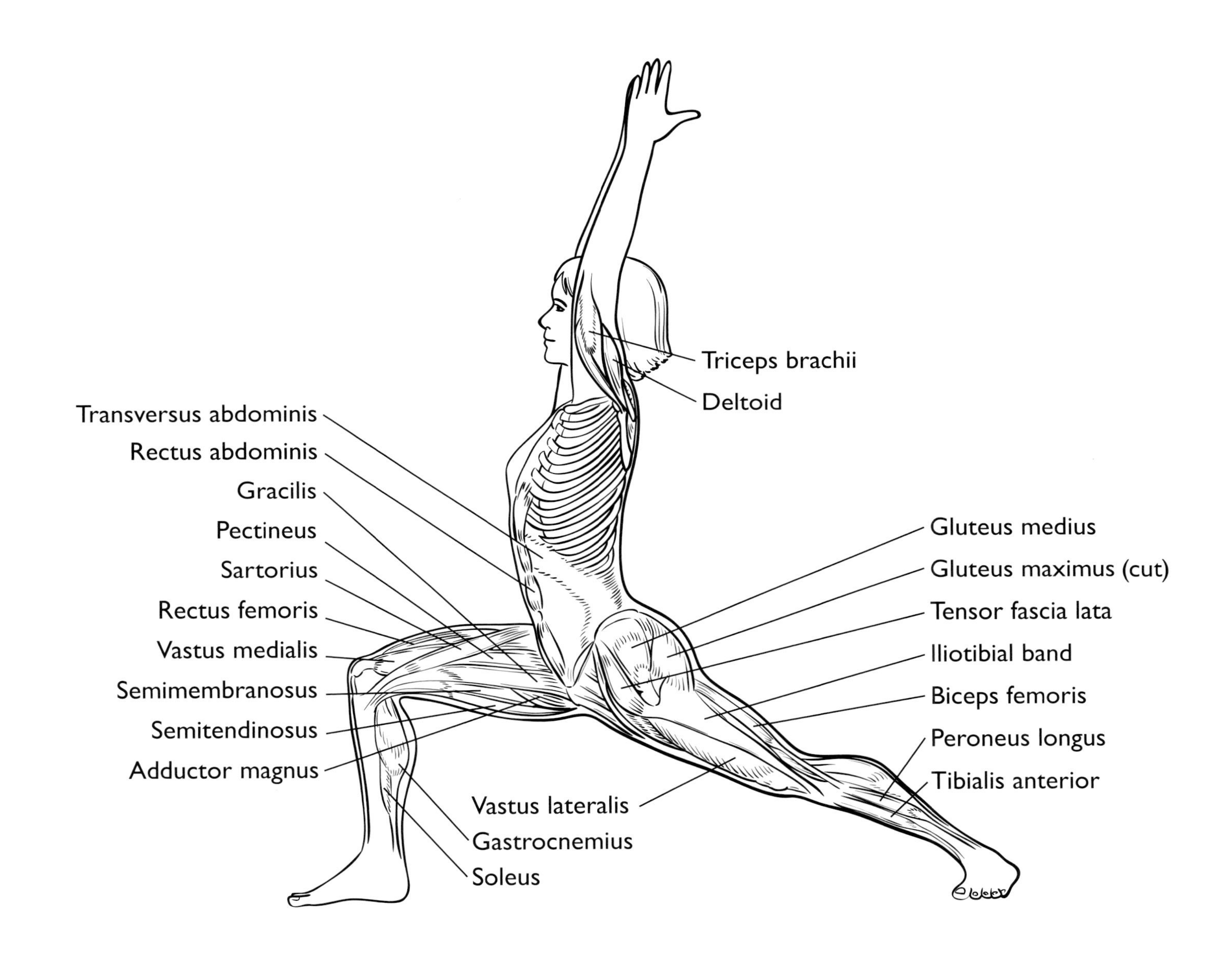

virabhadrasana I

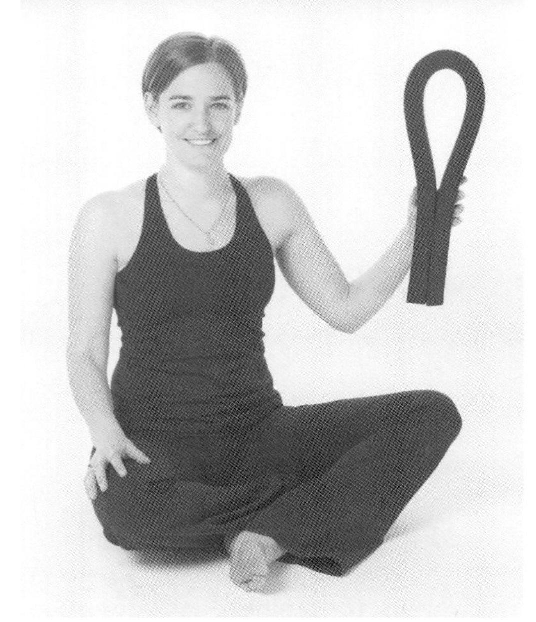

opening relaxation - 1

Virabhadrasana I

(Warrior I)

Consider your Anatomy: Virabhadrasana I, or Warrior I, can be challenging for people's knees, lower backs and, if the arms are raised, necks. To prevent these issues keep in mind the following key features: freedom through the rib cage, and front line of the body; pelvis square to the direction you are facing and think stability – hip abductors balanced with hip adductors balanced with the deeper pelvic muscles including the pelvic floor and external rotators. When you feel the subtly of this movement, Warrior will radiate from you. You'll feel much ease, space and lightness.

Move into Virabhadrasana I (both sides) and experience the pose. Where do you feel openness or freedom? Where is there release? Is there tension or discomfort? Where? Are you struggling? How?

Opening Relaxation: Spinal Strap Folded at T7-T8

1. Fold a spinal strap in half. Place the bottom of the fold at T7-T8 (where a bra strap would be).

2. Recline with the knees bent and feet planted on the ground.

3. The spinal strap runs upward along the spine from the fold at T7-T8 and supports the head. If there is discomfort in the back, elevate the buttocks with a folded blanket.

4. If you don't have a spinal strap or if the sensations caused by the pose are too intense, place a rolled yoga mat in the same position at T7-T8.

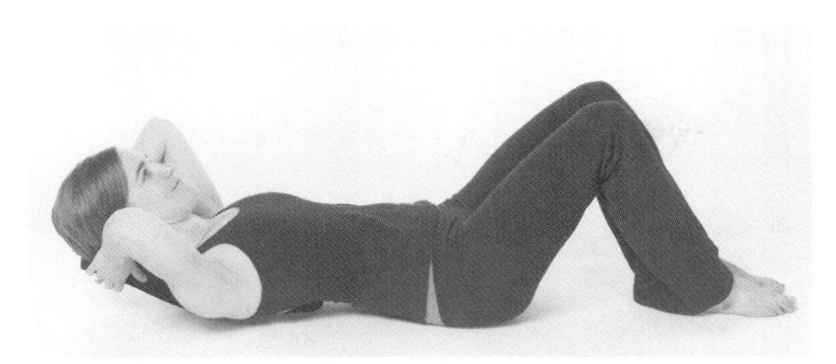
opening relaxation - 2

YOGA EXISTS IN THE WORLD

BECAUSE EVERYTHING IS LINKED.

—*Desikachar*

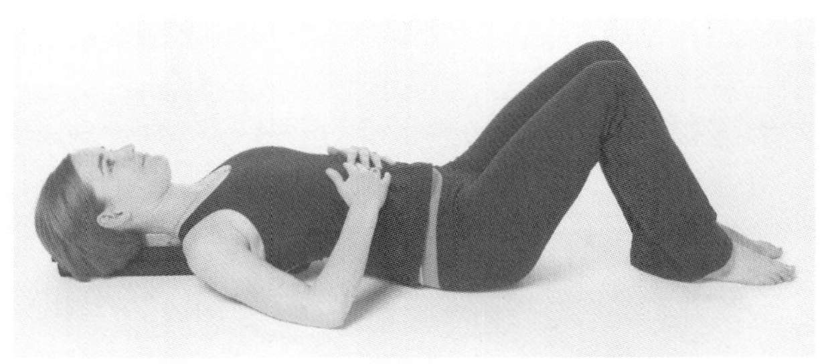
opening relaxation - 3

5. Relax in the position, and observe the sensations that arise. This might not be described as entirely comfortable! In your inhale imagine gently "expanding the chest" (where you have the greatest sensation of openness) and as you exhale imagine "letting go".

6. Be here for between one and five minutes. At any point, if pain occurs, the breath becomes haggard, or tension arises that can't be released with the breath and conscious softening, remove the black strap.

7. Remove the black strap and return to the reclined position without it. Notice the sensations in the front and back of the upper body. Is there a greater sense of space/openness in the chest? A greater connection of the upper back with the ground? How does it feel?

Reclined Shoulder Mobility with Spinal Strap

Return the black strap to its previous position at T7-T8 and recline once again with the knees bent and feet planted. Place your thumb-tips together, with fingers pointing to the sky.

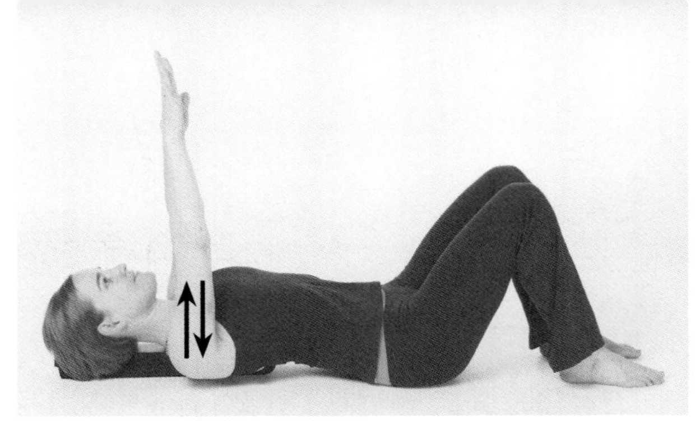

hands to the sky

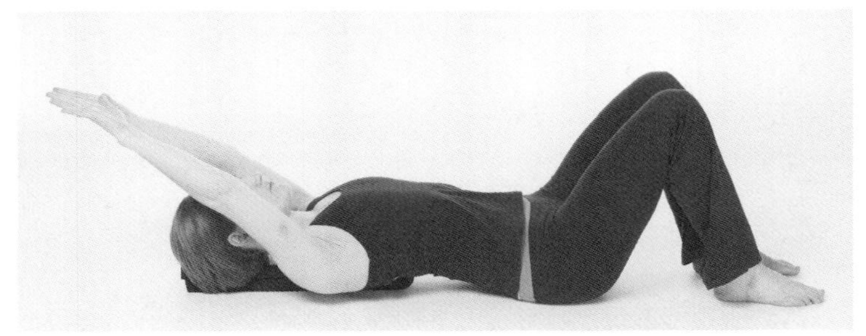

hands and arms overhead

Pullovers

(Hands to the Sky)

1. Elevate and straighten the arms so the wrists are directly over the shoulders. The arms are pointing straight up toward the sky (not back behind you!)

2. Gently draw the arm bones into the shoulder sockets and draw shoulder blades down toward the floor.

3. Moving with the breath, begin to slowly reach the arms toward the sky, and then draw them back down again. Repeat five to ten times.

Pullovers

(Hands and Arms Overhead)

1. Continuing to hold arm position as above (i.e. thumbtips touching), slowly arc the arms in the direction of over your head. Move with your breath.

2. The arms will float in a full half-circle. Move in your pain-free range of motion. The furthest you will go is arms alongside the ears. Be sure of the following:

- No clicking or pain.
- No backbending.

Repeat the arm arcs several times.

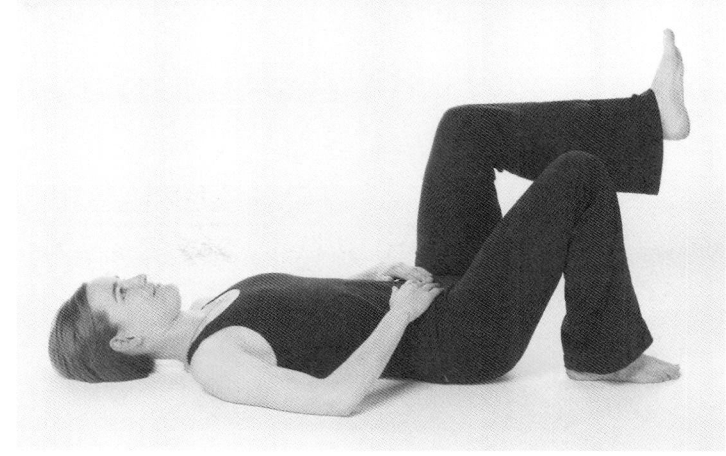

marching

DO YOUR PRACTICE AND ALL IS COMING.

—Sri K Patthabi Jois

Virabhadrasana I

(both sides)

Marching

1. Recline on the mat with both knees bent and the feet planted hip width apart. The pelvis and spine are neutral. The hands rest gently on the pelvis, palms down.

2. Gently lift the pelvic floor. Imagine flattening your belly without flattening your spine.

3. As you exhale, slowly float one bent leg up until the knee hovers over the hip and the lower leg is parallel to the floor.

4. As you inhale, slowly return the leg to its original position.

5. Change sides and repeat several times.

6. There should be no pelvic movement whatsoever – shifting, tucking – other than the continual, internal pelvic floor lift. The upper body remains completely at ease.

7. Repeat several times, breathing easily, and noticing the sensations that occur.

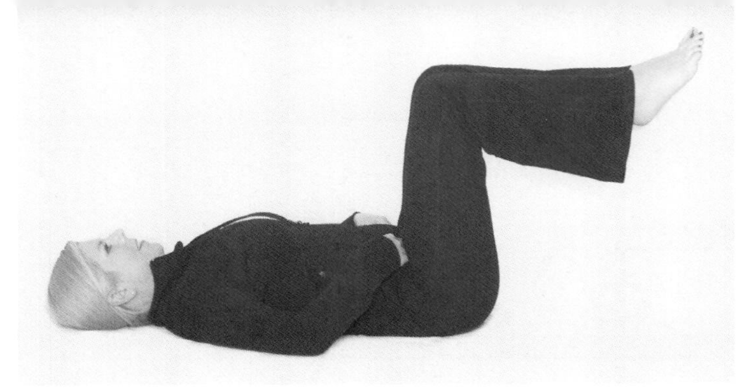

advanced marching - 1

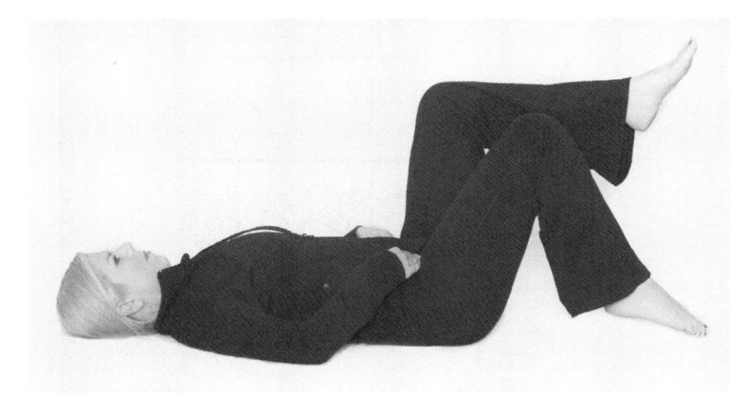

advanced marching - 2

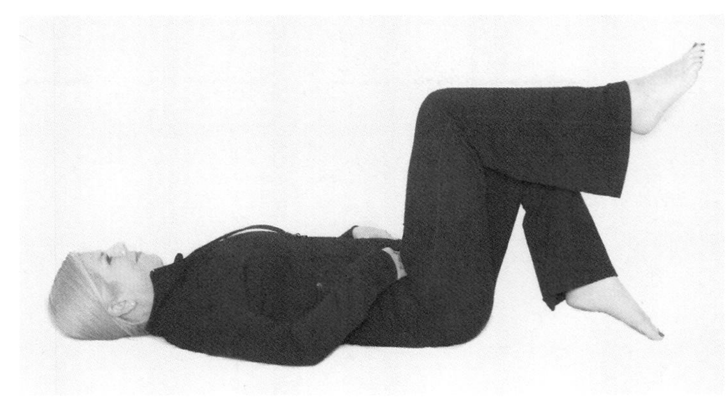

advanced marching - 3

Advanced Marching

1. Come into the same position as described above.

2. Gently lift the pelvic floor and flatten the belly without flattening the spine.

3. Slowly float both bent legs up until the knees hover above the hips and the lower legs are parallel to the floor or angled slightly upward.

4. Pause in place to ensure you are experiencing ease.

5. As you inhale, slowly dip one bent leg toward the ground, touching the tips of the toes lightly to floor as though you're testing the water. As you exhale, gently lift the leg back into place.

6. Change sides and repeat several times.

7. As above, there should be no pelvic movement whatsoever – shifting, tucking – other than the continual, internal pelvic floor lift. The upper body remains completely at ease. Sometimes there is a tendency to bring the knees in toward the chest. Don't let them. You'll work more effectively if the knees hover over the hips, instead of drawing them in closer to the chest.

8. Repeat several times, breathing easily, and noticing the sensations that occur.

Calf Stretch at Wall

1. Stand facing the wall with the feet hip width apart.

2. Keep the right foot facing forward on the floor right at the edge of the wall, and take a medium step back with the left foot.

3. The hips should be equidistant to both the floor and wall.

4. The hands are flat on the wall in front of the chest, shoulder width apart. Keep the upper body relaxed.

5. Slowly start to bend the right knee forward, keeping the left heel connected with the ground, until you feel a stretch.

6. Press down into the left heel and imagine drawing energy from the earth, up into the arch of the left foot, and up into the inner thigh.

7. Breathe and observe the sensations.

8. If more intensity is required, step slightly further back with the left foot keeping the toes pointing forward.

9. Pause and come into Tadasana. Observe the sensations, left and right.

Change sides.

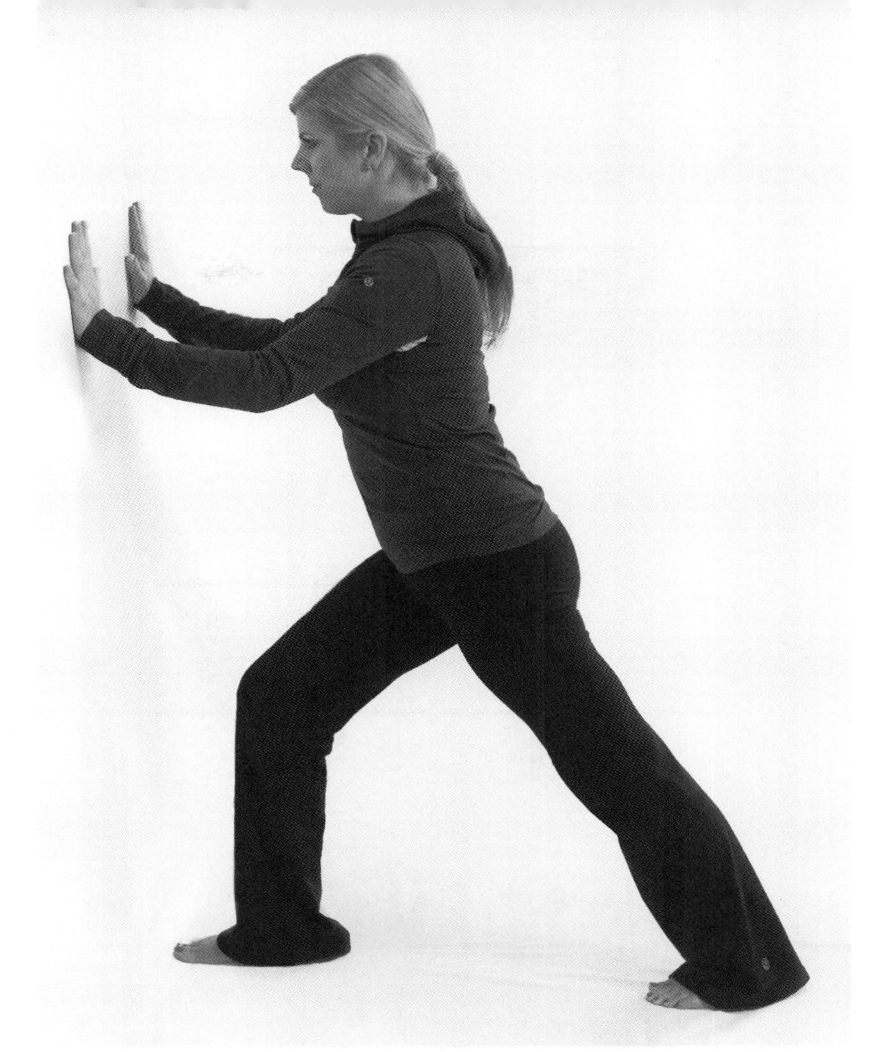

calf stretch at wall

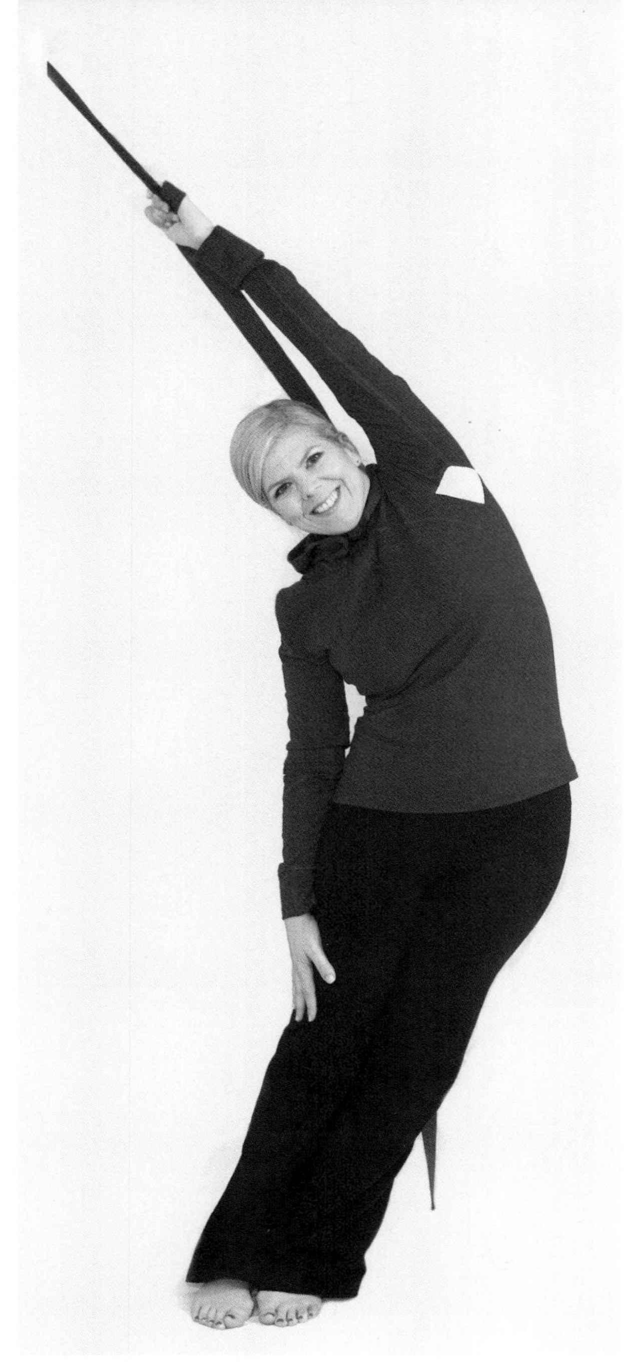
side bend with strap over door

❁ *Virabhadrasana I*

(both sides)

Side Bend with Strap Over Door

1. Place the top end of a strap over the top of a door and close the door, pulling the strap taught.

2. Stand perpendicular to the wall and take the arm that's farthest from the door overhead.

3. Loop the strap around the hand a couple of times until it's stable and the strap won't slide when you pull away from the wall.

4. Holding the strap, start to lean the body away from the door, leading with the hips. The sensations in the side body will probably differ depending on what part of the body presses away from the wall. Experiment with pressing out into the hips, waist, ribs and underarm. The strap can feel tight around the hand. Feel free to pause and relax the hand periodically, if necessary.

Release the arm and come into Tadasana. Observe the sensations left and right.

Change sides.

Virabhadrasana I

(both sides)

Wall Sit with Block

1. Stand with the back against a wall, feet hip width apart.

2. As you step the feet forward, slowly slide the back down the wall until simulating a seated position.

3. The lower you go, the more challenging this will be! Take care to not surpass your edge. (To ensure you do not surpass your edge find a position you can easily be in for 30 minutes. You won't be in this for 30 minutes, however, by following this guideline, you will know you are in the right place for your body.)

4. Place a block between the thighs one inch from your pubic bone and ensure that the knees are positioned comfortably over the ankles. (Instead of using blocks between the thighs, you can tie a strap around the thighs and press out gently. Try both, and see which gives you more lightness and ease.)

5. Let the arms hang easily at the sides of the body, with the shoulders relaxed and the spine neutral.

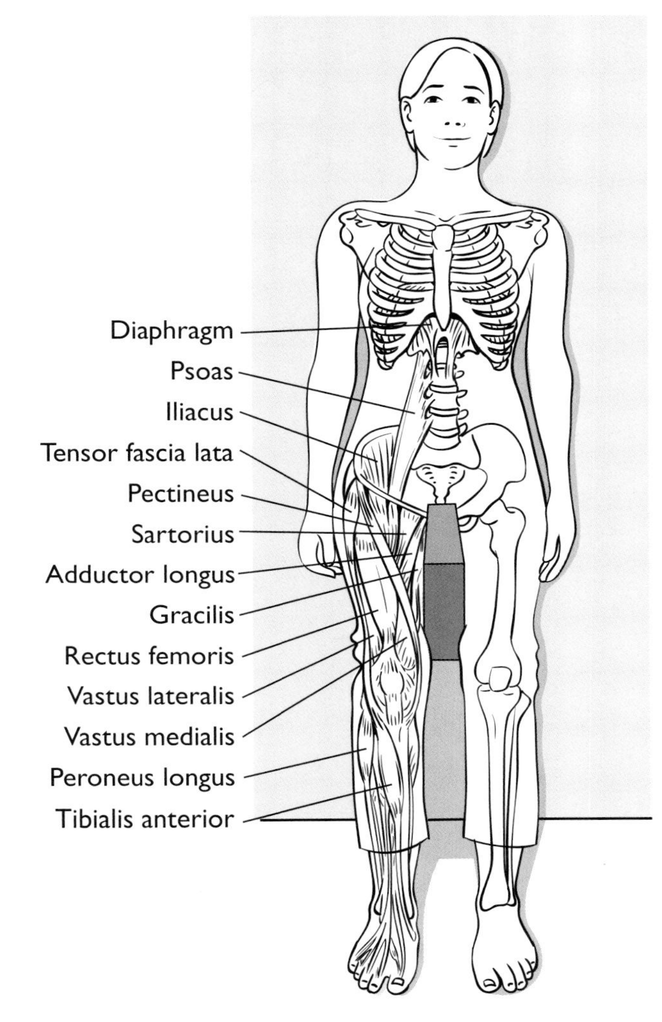

wall sit with block

6. Breathe easily in place and observe the sensations.

7. To come out of the pose, slowly slide the back up the wall. Thrusting yourself away from the wall can strain the back, so be sure to be mindful during the dismount.

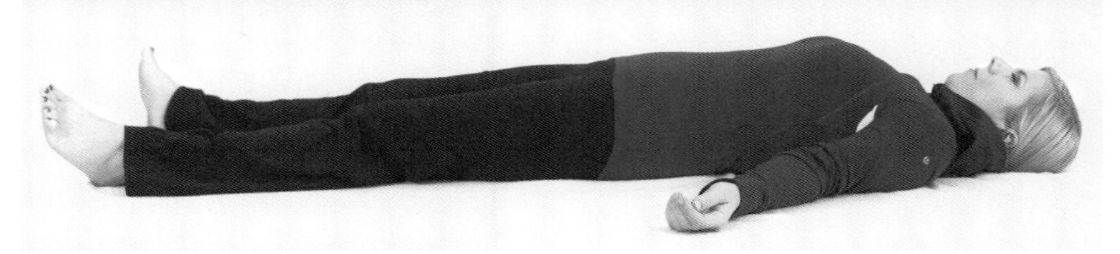

savasana

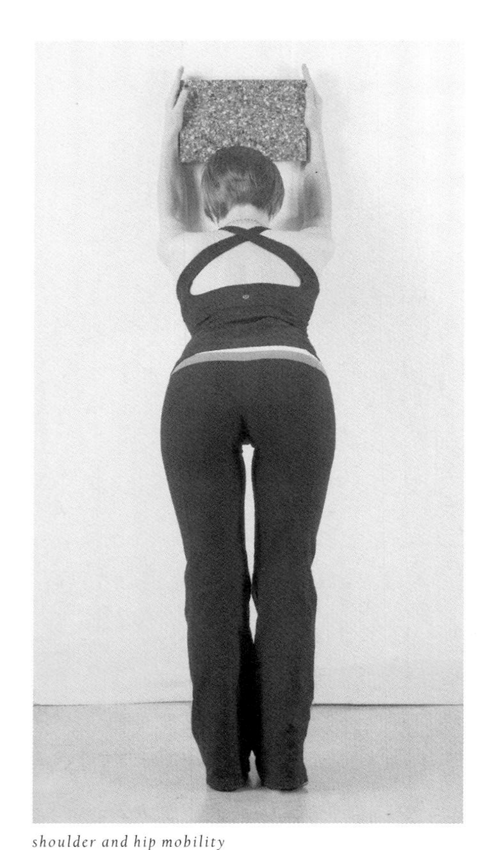

shoulder and hip mobility

Shoulder and Hip Mobility

1. Press the hands into a block that's turned horizontally, so that they're roughly shoulder width apart.

2. Face the wall and place the forearms on it, moving the hips back until they're over the ankles.

3. The spine is neutral and pelvis is stable.

4. The shoulders are stable and strong and the arm bones are drawn into their shoulder sockets.

5. Breathe and observe.

6. This pose can also be done with the fingers interlaced and the elbows shoulder width apart.

Virabhadrasana I

(both sides)

With your right foot forward, place your right hand on the outside of your right thigh. Gently press the thigh into your hand. Notice what happens at your ankle, knee, and hip. If you tend to be a pronator, you will see your ankle shift position and your knee alignment change. Press as much as you need to have appropriate alignment for your body.

Savasana

As you lay back in Savasana, feel the strength in your legs, the openness in your pelvis, chest and arms. Next, feel the back of your head and spine. Drink in this sense of strength and openness. Enjoy!

Questions to consider:
How did my body feel in the various positions? Which did it enjoy, if so why? If not, why not? How did the Side Bend impact Virabhadrasana I? Am I able to differentiate between the feelings on opposites sides of my body? How does it feel to slow down and focus inward? What differences, subtle or obvious, can I feel in the pose from the first to the last instance? Do I think that I have a better awareness of the movement required to access this pose safely and effectively in my practice? Which exercise had the greatest impact, and why?

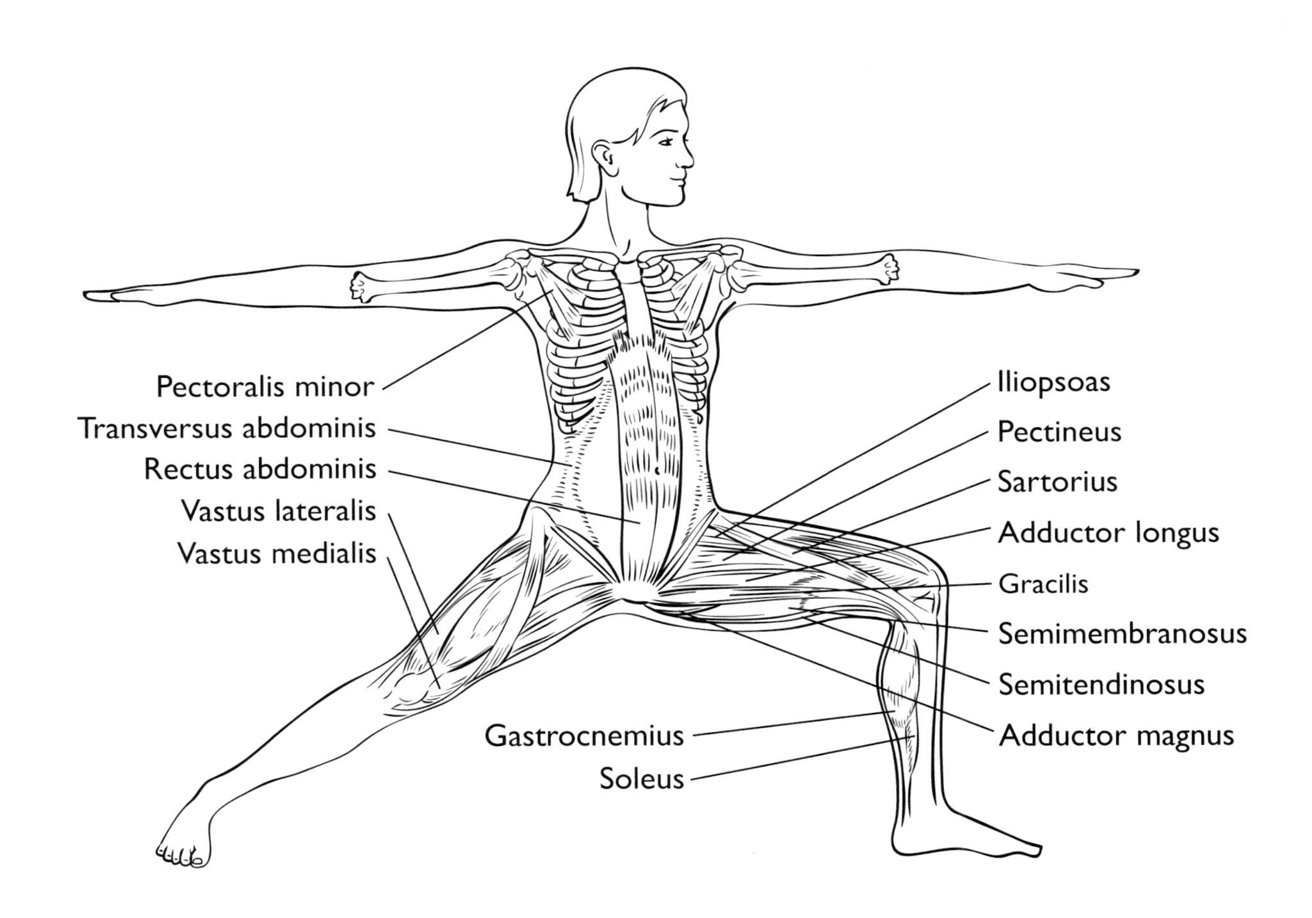

virabhadrasana II

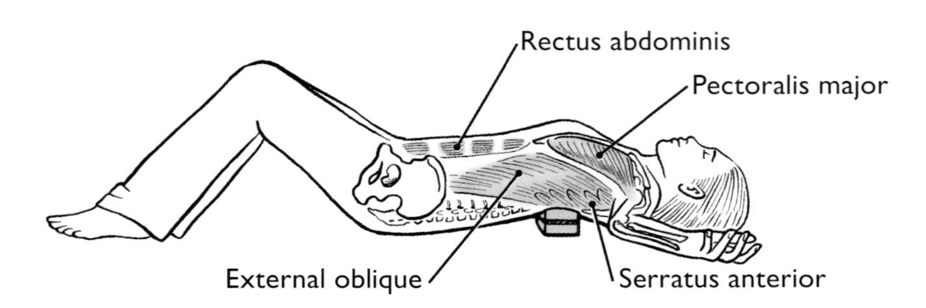

folded black strap across T7-T8

Virabhadrasana II

(Warrior II)

Consider your Anatomy: Virabhadrasana II, or Warrior II, flows organically from Virabhadrasana I, or Warrior I, where the release and openness in the rib cage and thoracic spine connects with new leg and pelvis positions. If there is shortness or tightness through the hips preventing pure motion, leg, pelvic and spinal movement can become jammed, which tends to result in compensating elsewhere like the knees, sacroiliac joints, or further up the spine.

Ask the students to come into Virabhadrasana II (both sides) and experience the pose. Where do you feel open, free? Is there tension or discomfort? Where? Are you struggling? How?

Opening Relaxation: Folded Spinal Strap Across T7-T8

1. Fold a spinal strap in half. Place the strap horizontally across the back at T7-T8 (where a bra strap would be).

2. Slowly recline with the knees bent and feet planted on the ground.

3. As you recline, take care to maintain the connection between the ribs and top of the pelvis. If there is discomfort in the back, elevate the buttocks with a folded blanket.

4. If you don't have a spinal strap or if the sensations caused by the pose are too intense, place a rolled yoga mat in the same position at T7-T8.

5. Relax in the position, and observe the sensations that arise. This might not be entirely comfortable! Imagine gently "expanding the chest" (where you have the greatest sensation of openness) as you inhale and "letting go" as you exhale.

6. Stay in the position for one to five minutes. At any point, if pain occurs, or the breath becomes haggard, or tension arises that can't be released with the breath and conscious softening, remove the black strap.

7. When you are ready to come out, remove the black strap and return to the reclined position without it.

8. Notice the sensations in the front and back of the upper body. Is there a greater sense of space/ openness in the chest? A greater connection of the upper back with the ground? How does it feel?

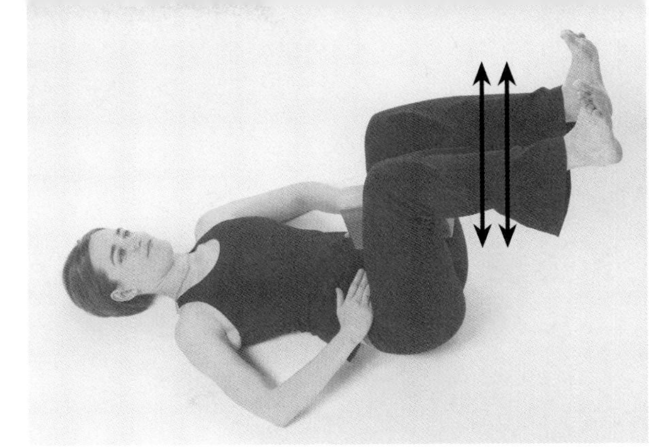

tick tocks

֍ *Virabhadrasana II*

(both sides)

Tick Tocks

1. Recline on the mat with both knees bent and the feet planted hip width apart. The pelvis and spine are neutral. The hands rest gently on the pelvis, palms down.

2. Gently lift the pelvic floor and flatten your belly without flattening your spine.

3. Place a block between the thighs. Slowly float both bent legs up until the knees hover above the hips and the lower legs are parallel to the floor.

4. Pause in place to ensure the pelvis, spine and the upper body are at ease.

5. Maintaining this position, gently "Tick Tock" the legs a few inches to the left and right. Continue this subtle moment from side to side with the legs, breathing easily, and noticing the sensations that occur.

6. Take a break and relax as required.

7. Avoid the temptation to bring the knees in toward the chest. You'll work more effectively if the knees hover over the hips, instead of drawing them in closer to the chest, and you'll be in a position for better gains in strength and stability.

8. Remember to keep your jaw, mouth, lips and eyes relaxed. You'll feel more in your abdomen.

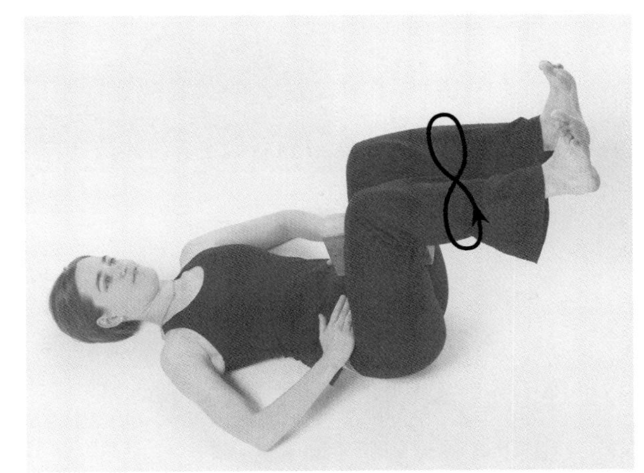

figure 8

Figure 8

1. The set-up for this exercise is exactly the same as above, with the block between the knees and the knees hovering above the hips.

2. Instead of "Tick Tock", though, draw small figure 8's with the knees. Repeat several times and then change the direction of the figure 8's.

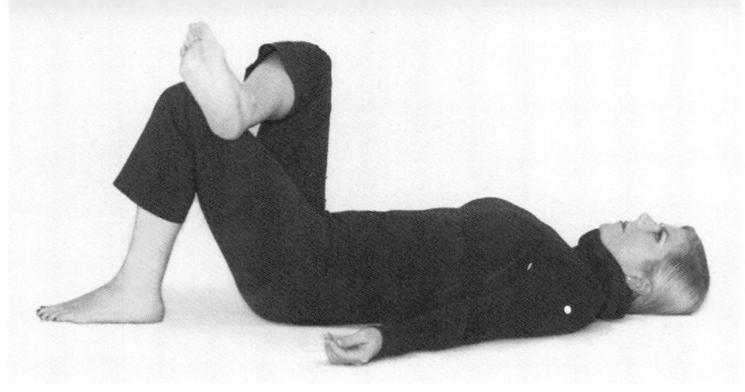

ankle to knee, then twist - 1

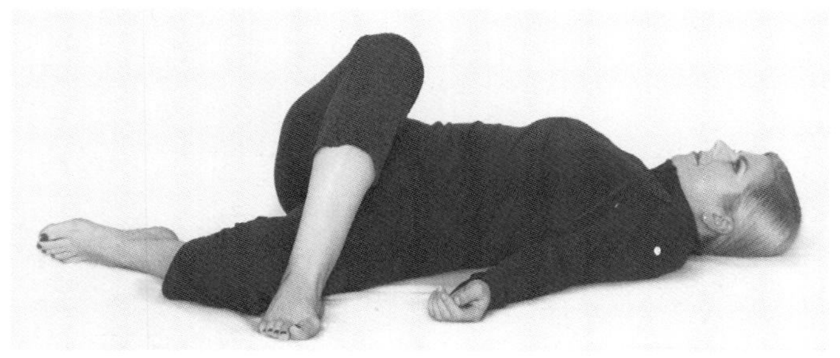

ankle to knee, then twist - 2

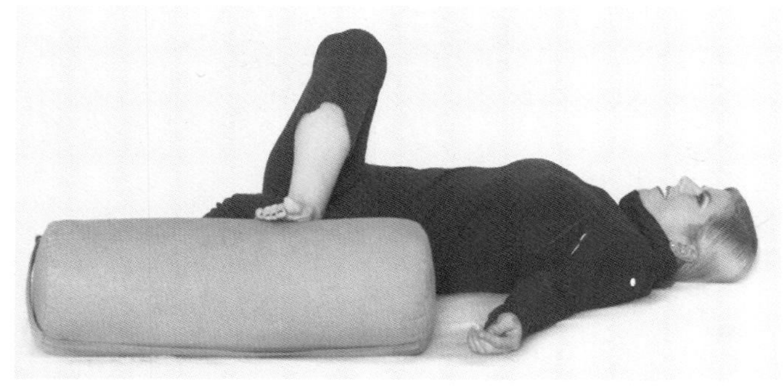

ankle to knee, then twist - modification

Ankle to Knee, Then Twist

1. Recline with the knees bent and feet planted on the ground.

2. Slowly cross the right ankle onto the left knee, without displacing or shifting the pelvis as you come into position.

3. Begin to lower the legs to the left, without either shifting the position of the lower foot on the floor or the upper ankle on the knee.

4. Ideally, the right knee points straight up to the sky while the right foot is supported above the floor on a bolster or folded blanket. (If your body feels good, allow the foot to come to the floor.)

5. The arms are about 45 degrees away from the body, with the palms facing up, the shoulders comfortable. The gaze is to the sky.

6. Imagine the entire right side of the pelvis sinking into the ground. Imagine the head of the right femur sinking back into its hip socket.

7. Relinquish any tension in the legs, hips, buttocks and lower back. Observe the sensations. Breathe into the stretch and settle for a few minutes.

Sometimes in this pose, "hip jigging" occurs, where when twisting left, the left pelvis slides up to the left ribs, shortening that side. Allow the twist to be pure. Don't let the hips jig.

8. Slowly come out of the pose and observe the sensations in the body. Compare both side of the pelvis and lower back.

Change sides.

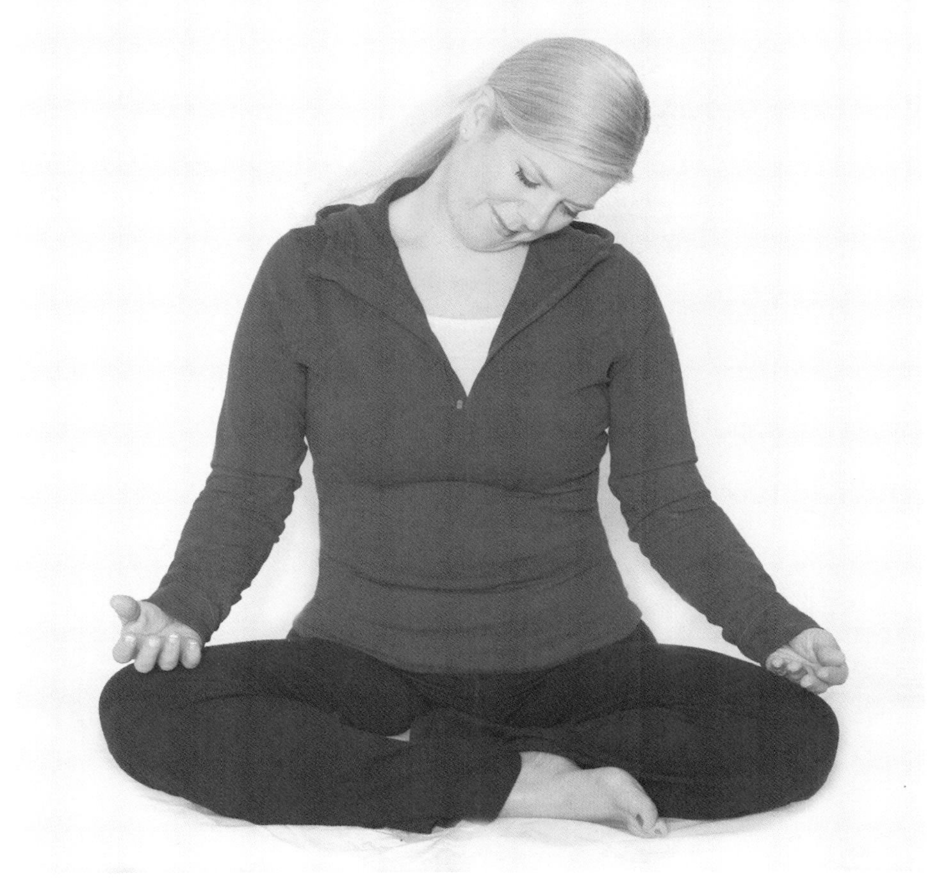

neck rolls

❁ *Virabhadrasana II*

(both sides)

Neck Rolls

1. Assume a comfortable seated position. Imagine creating length through both the back and front of the neck as you slowly lower the chin toward the chest.

2. Relax in place for a few breaths.

3. Slowly start to roll the head to the left until the left ear comes to the left shoulder. Keep the shoulders relaxed and the head heavy, throughout.

4. Slowly roll the head down again, arcing the chin across the chest until the right ear comes to the right shoulder.

5. Repeat the movement several times and notice what you feel. Pause in these places and breathe.

6. To come out of the movement, slowly roll the chin back down to the centre of the chest and lift the head back up to centre. Pause and breathe comfortably, noticing the sensations.

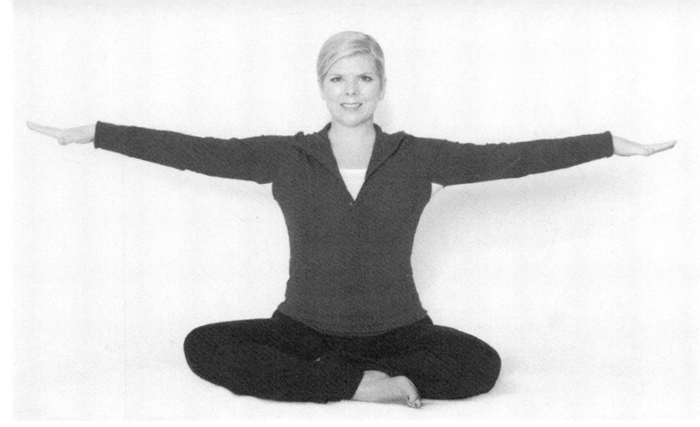

arm stretch and strengtheners - 1

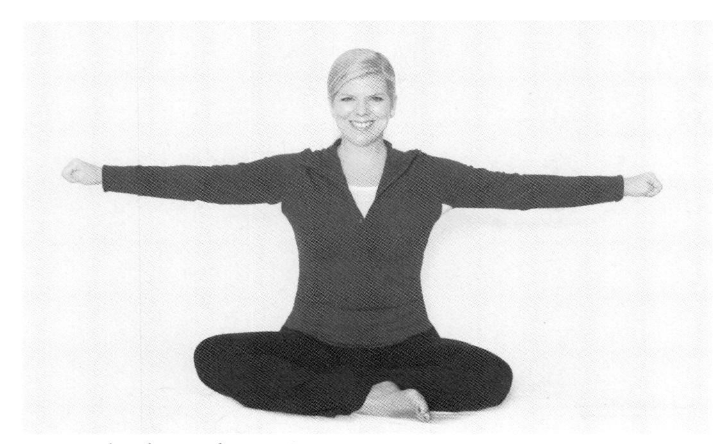

arm stretch and strengtheners - 2

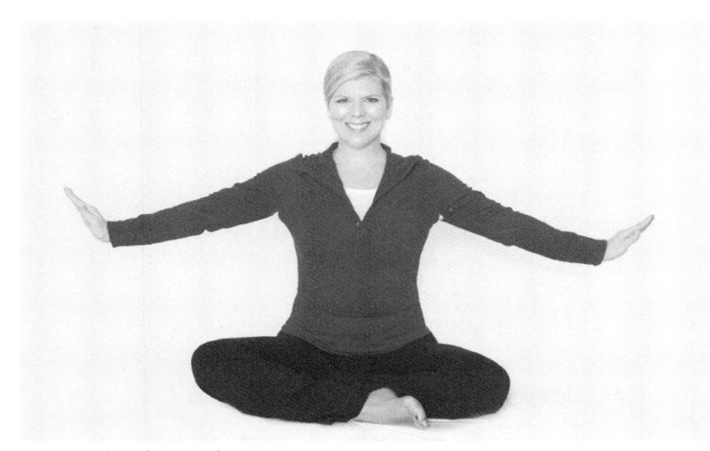

arm stretch and strengtheners - 3

Arm Stretch & Strengtheners

1. Sit comfortably with the arms at the sides.

2. Keeping the shoulders down and relaxed, press out with both palms, the fingers and thumbs side by side (not spread out).

3. Slowly start to lift the arms out and away from the body until you feel a stretch. Pause and breathe.

4. If the stretch is not too intense, the arms can be raised as high as shoulder height above the ground.

5. Continue to breathe easy and observe. If tingling or numbness occur, take a break.

6. With the arms still out at shoulder height, draw the hands into fists and then open the fingers.

7. Repeat this opening and closing motion with the hands, keeping the shoulders relaxed. Repeat five to ten times and then relax the arms back down at the sides, noticing the changing sensations.

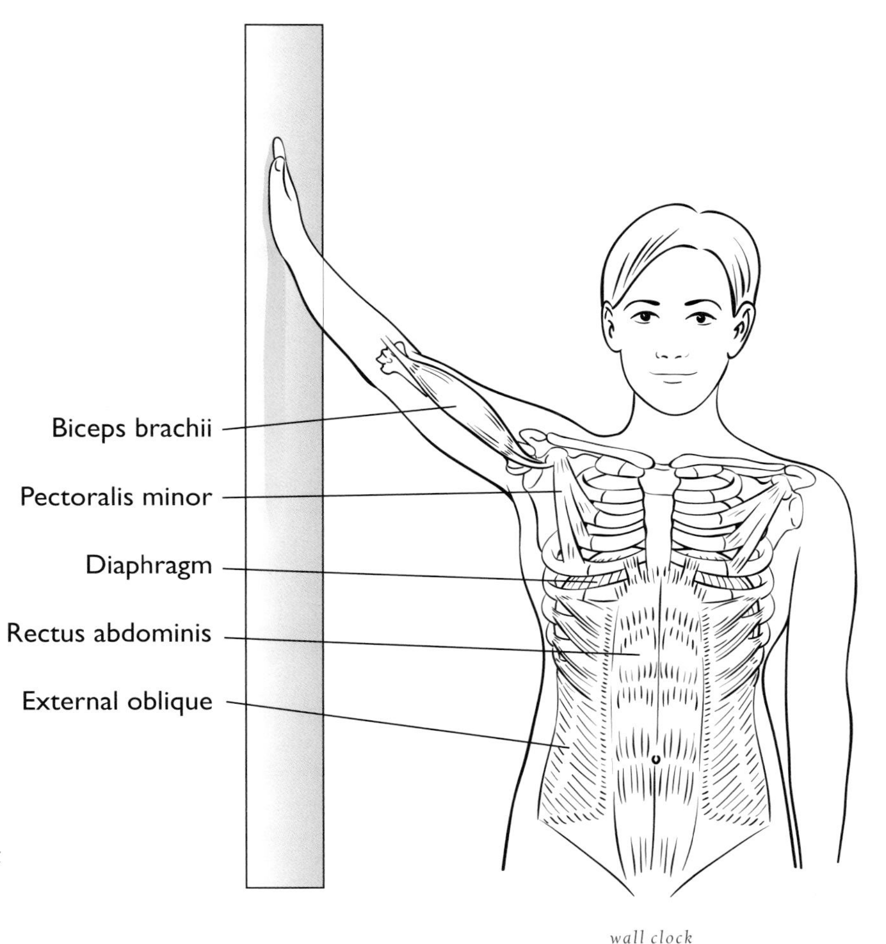

wall clock

Wall Clock

1. Stand perpendicular to the wall with the right side of the body closest to the wall.

2. Take the right arm straight up along wall with the palm flat and the arm straight. If there is any tension or lifting whatsoever in the right shoulder, step away from the wall and lower the arm as necessary, keeping the palm flat and connected.

3. Stand in a balanced way, far enough away from the wall so that the shoulders both stay down and tension-free.

4. The right arm is now at 12 o'clock. If there are sensations of stretching, maintain this position and breathe in place. If not, slowly take the hand/arm back to 1 o'clock. The chest faces forward, throughout. The right shoulder and chest should not rotate as the arm comes back.

5. Let the shoulders be relaxed and free of gripping. Stay in the pose and breathe easily observing the sensations. If tingling or numbness occur, take a break until it subsides.

6. Lower the arm after a minute or two (assuming there was no pain, tingling or numbness) and stand in Tadasana observing the sensations in both the left and right side.

Change sides.

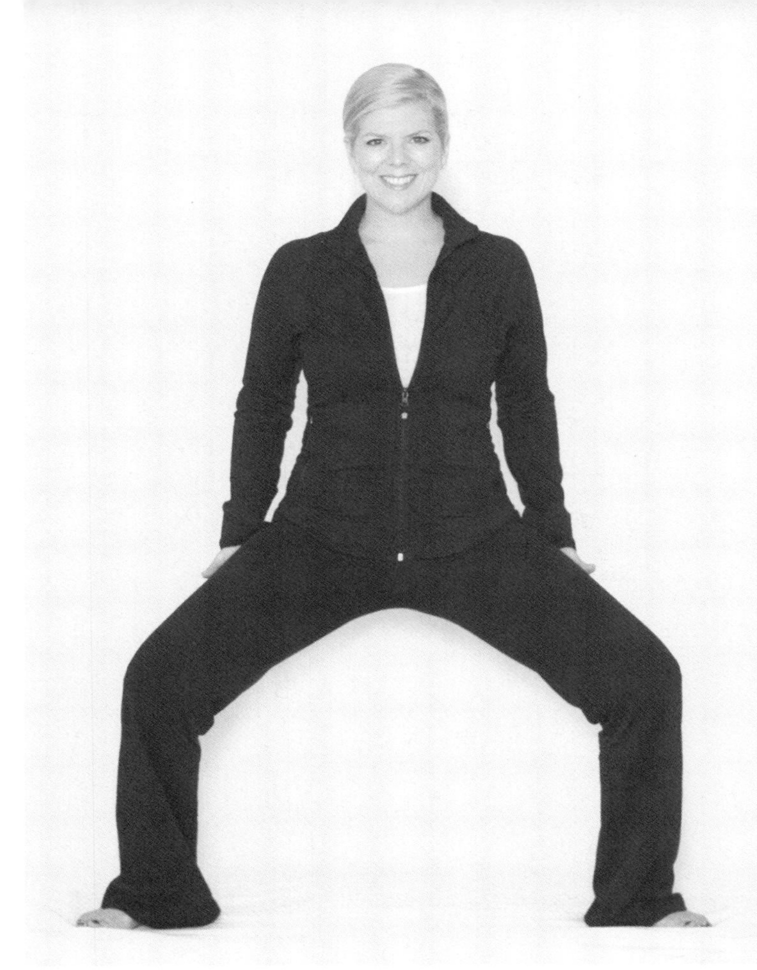

goddess pose

Virabhadrasana II

(both sides)

Goddess Pose

1. Stand on the mat with the legs about a leg-length apart.

2. Angle the feet outward about 45 degrees. Keeping the pelvis neutral, slowly bend the knees, encouraging them to move/roll outward.

3. Come to your comfortable edge.

4. Taking care to keep the pelvis and spine neutral, place the hands on the upper, outer thighs/hips and gently press into them. Notice if this changes the experience of the pose. How?

5. Continue to observe as you stay in the pose for several breaths.

Warrior Series at Wall

1. Place the feet in a Virabhadrasana II stance at the wall with the right foot pointing forward and the back foot angled slightly inward. The front foot should be several inches away from the wall.

2. As you bend the front knee forward over the ankle, place a block in between the upper, outer right thigh and the wall. There should be enough space between the foot and the wall so that you're comfortable against the block and you're not supporting yourself by leaning against the wall.

3. Press the right upper leg gently into the block. Do not allow the right knee to collapse in, away from the wall — it stays aligned with the hip and ankle.

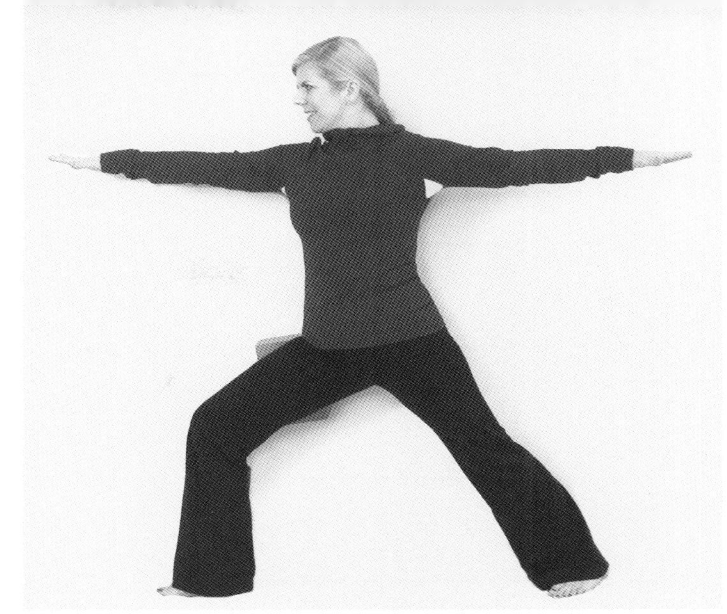

warrior series at wall - 1

4. With the chest open, and the collar bones broad, elevate the arms to shoulder height, coming into Virabhadrasana II.

5. If it's not uncomfortable for the neck, take the gaze forward, beyond the right hand. Note: There should not be any strain, stretch or pain in the back foot or ankle. If this occurs, step this foot a little further away from the wall.

6. Notice if this variation of the pose feels different from your usual Virabhadrasana II. Hold for several breaths, observing.

7. Keeping the legs solidly in place, slowly lift the right arm up to the sky (palm facing back behind you), as the left hand lowers lightly onto the left thigh. Hold this position for several breaths, observing.

8. Moving with the breath, and still keeping the legs in place, return to Virabhadrasana II. Breathe easily as you repeat several times.

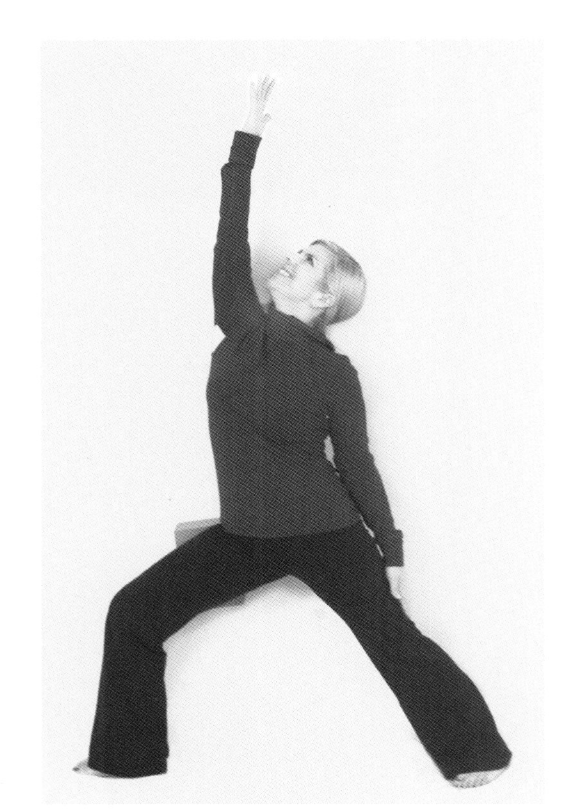

warrior series at wall - 2

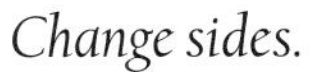

Change sides.

WITH OUR BREATH,

WE KEEP THE PLANET FROM BECOMING A DESERT.

—*Veronique Vienne*

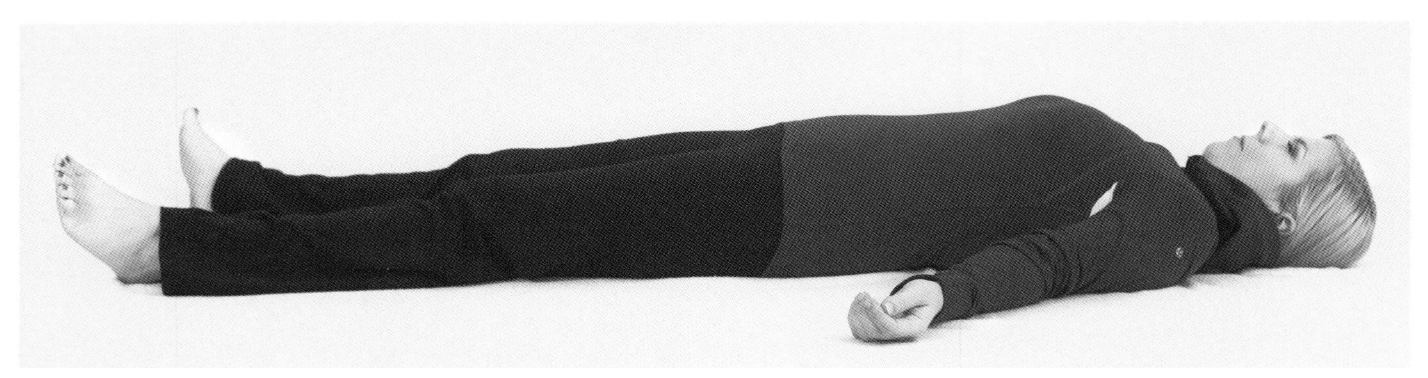

savasana

Savasana

On your back, feel the sensations of your body. Fee the breath move through your rib cage with each inhale and exhale. Bring your awareness to the outer ribs and armpits and feel the breath moving. Imagine breathing through your armpits. After several breaths, imagine breathing through your groins. Next, imagine breathing through your feet. Connect all three points and feel the breath through your entire body.

Questions to consider:
How did my body feel in the various positions? Which did it enjoy, if so why? If not, why not? Did my hips jig? Did my stability, mobility and strength improve? Was I able to feel more? Am I able to differentiate between the feelings on opposites sides of my body? How does it feel to slow down and focus inward? What differences, subtle or obvious, can I feel in the pose from the first to the last instance? Do I think that I have a better awareness of the movement required to access this pose safely and effectively in my practice? Which exercise had the greatest impact, and why?

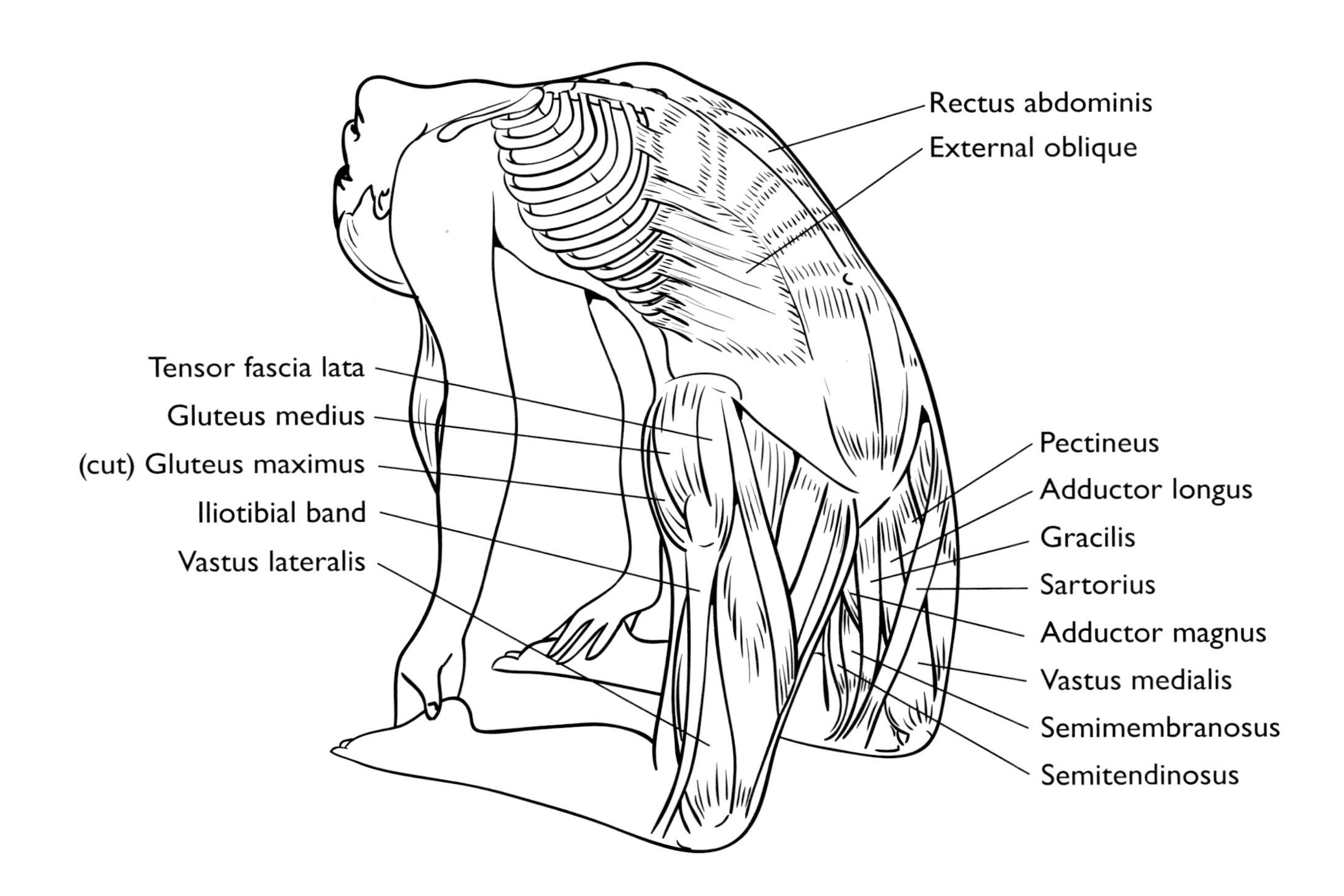
Rectus abdominis
External oblique
Tensor fascia lata
Gluteus medius
(cut) Gluteus maximus
Iliotibial band
Vastus lateralis
Pectineus
Adductor longus
Gracilis
Sartorius
Adductor magnus
Vastus medialis
Semimembranosus
Semitendinosus

ustrasana

ASANA BRINGS STEADINESS, HEALTH AND LIGHTNESS OF LIMB.

A STEADY AND PLEASANT POSTURE PRODUCES MENTAL EQUILIBRIUM AND PREVENTS FICKLENESS OF MIND.

ASANAS ARE NOT MERELY GYMNASTICS EXERCISES; THEY ARE POSTURES.

—BKS Iyengar

Ustrasana

(Camel Pose)

Consider your Anatomy: Ustrasana, or Camel Pose, is a traction back bend, which moves you backward with gravity. It asks for an extension through the spine and hips that is smooth and open. This pose specifically requests a release of the myofascia of quadriceps, hip flexors, rectus abdominis, the obliques bilaterally, pectoralis major and minor, and neck flexors. There is a trick to this occurring — because this back bend moves with gravity, all of these muscles will be also eccentrically contracting to mediate the motion. It is important to easily breathe while engaging your deep core from the feet to the skull, as well as stability through your hip abductors so that smooth movement occurs.

Remember, if there is excessive movement at T12, L1, L2, L3, L4 or L5 or if there is highly limited movement at T4, T5, T6, T7 or T8, there will be an opportunity to jam in the neck, flare out the ribs, compress at the L5-S1 junction or harm the sacro-iliac joints.

Move into Ustrasana or modified Ustrasana (see below) and experience the pose. Where do you feel open and free? Where? Is there tension or discomfort? Where? Are you struggling? How?

This pose is often a challenge for even seasoned yogis. I recommend the following: Kneeling upright, with knees hip width apart, make fists and place them on either side of the back of the pelvis, encouraging openness in this region. Try to keep the heads of the femurs overtop of the knees. With the pelvic floor lifted, and belly gently contracted, extend upward through the spine. Only if it is available, come into a back bend.

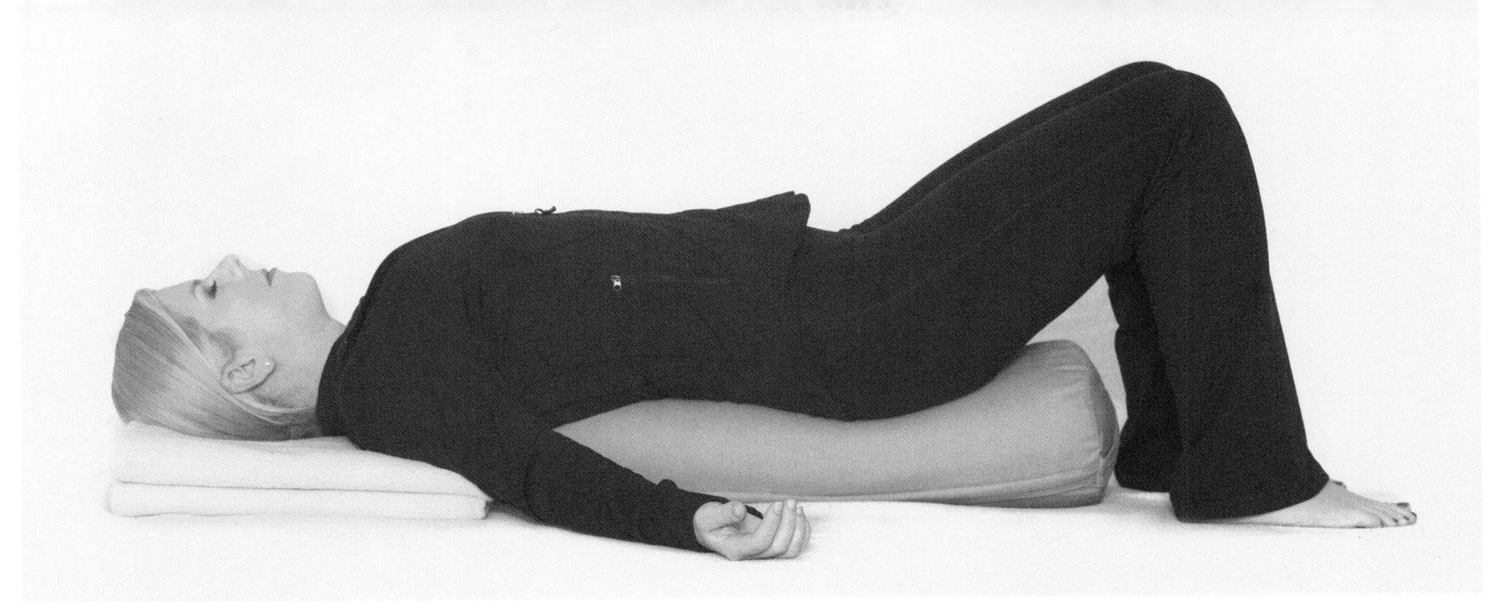

recline on bolster

Opening Relaxation: Recline on Bolster

1. Place a bolster vertically along the mat.

2. With the knees bent and the feet planted on the ground, sit toward the front of the bolster and lower the back onto it so that the top edge of the bolster is at T7-T8.

3. Support the shoulders and head as necessary with folded blankets.

Note: This backbend can be really intense for some people. If it's too intense, elevate the feet with yoga blocks, or support with more blankets as required. If this doesn't help, use the spinal strip and its modifications.

4. Relax and breathe for several minutes, noticing the sensations and the breath.

Ustrasana or Modified Ustrasana

Roll Out Chest and Underarms with Tennis Ball at the Wall

1. Stand facing the wall and place a tennis ball at the upper, outer chest, between the collarbones and underarm.

2. Roll gently and experience what you feel.

3. If you discover places that feel particularly tight, pause in place and breathe into the tightness.

PEOPLE SOMETIMES ASK ME WHAT DIFFERENCE PRACTICE HAS MADE IN MY LIFE.

THE ANSWER IS IT'S CHANGED EVERYTHING FOR ME. AND, IN A FUNNY WAY, IT'S CHANGED NOTHING.

—*Lama Surya Das*

4. Move slowly left and right, up and down, exploring the entire chest region.

5. We call these areas sweet spots because it is soooo sweet when they let go and release. To help with this, relax your jaw, eyes, toes and your pelvic floor.

6. Pause with both arms relaxed at the sides of the body and notice if there are different sensations in the left and right side.

7. Turn the body so that the underarm is facing the wall. Elevate the same arm and place ball at the underarm.

8. Apply slight pressure and observe what you feel. If you discover places that feel particularly tight, pause in place and breathe.

9. Move slowly left and right, up and down, exploring the entire underarm region.

10. Pause with both arms relaxed at the sides of the body and notice if the sensations have changed.

11. Roll out the other side of the body — both the chest and underarm areas.

12. Pause with both arms relaxed at the sides of the body and notice the sensations.

Ustrasana *or* Modified Ustrasana

As you practice your Camel or modified Camel, try adding a block between the thighs one inch from the pubic bone. This will help engage the inner thighs and support your core line. You can also tie a strap around your thighs, mid-thigh height and gently press into the strap. Which do you like better?

Engage your feet. By gently pressing the top of the foot just behind the big toe and just behind the pinky toe you may also feel a slight lift leading to greater ease in this back bend.

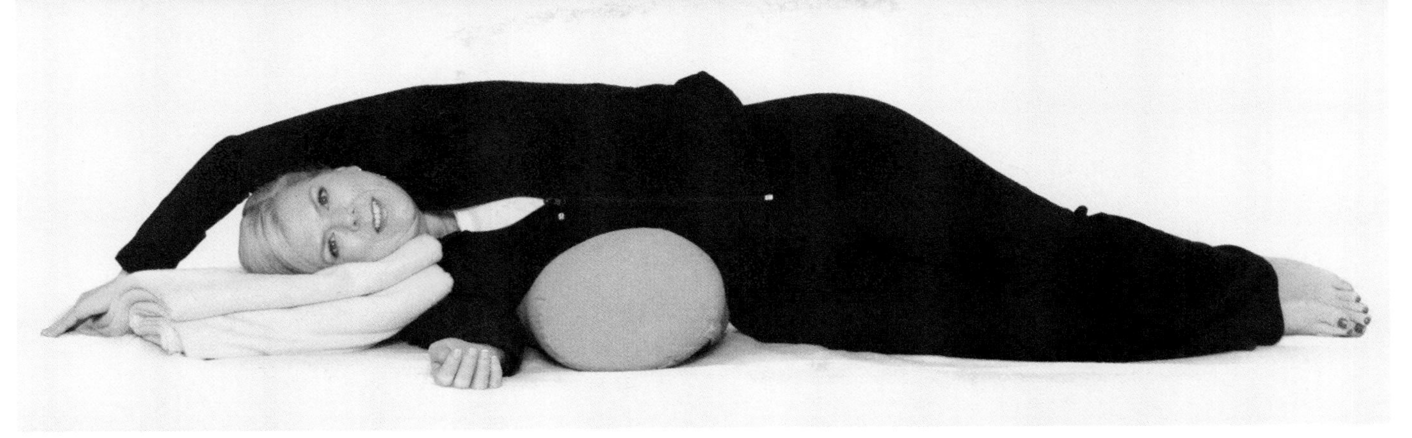

side stretch over bolster

Side Stretch Over Bolster

1. Lie on one side over a bolster that's placed horizontally on the mat. The bolster supports the rib cage, and the bottom hip is on the ground.

2. The shoulders and head will be on the other side of the bolster, and should be supported with blankets, as necessary.

3. Place the top hand on the top hip, palm facing up.

4. Slowly lift the arm in an arc toward the ceiling until it comes alongside the ear. Notice the sensations along the side of the body closest to the sky.

5. If this is too intense, support the bottom hip with a folded blanket. If more intensity is desired, you have several options:

- Extend the legs toward the bottom of the mat until they are straight.
- Rotate the top arm/shoulder slightly forward or backward until the sensations deepen.
- Elevate the bolster by placing a folded blanket(s) on top of it.

6. Breathe and relax in place. On each inhale, imagine gently inflating the place where the stretch occurs.

Change sides.

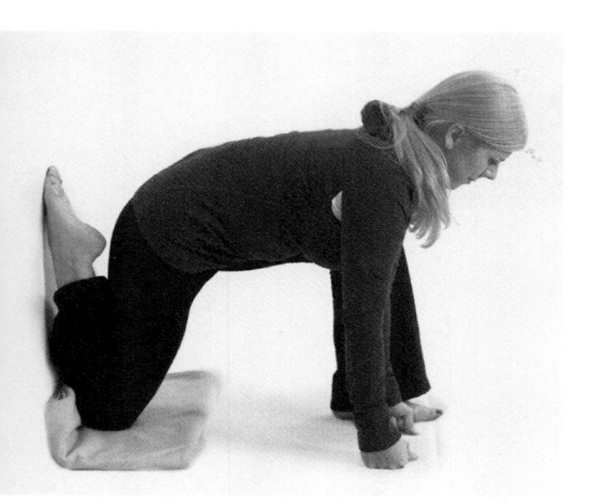
quad stretch series at the wall - 1

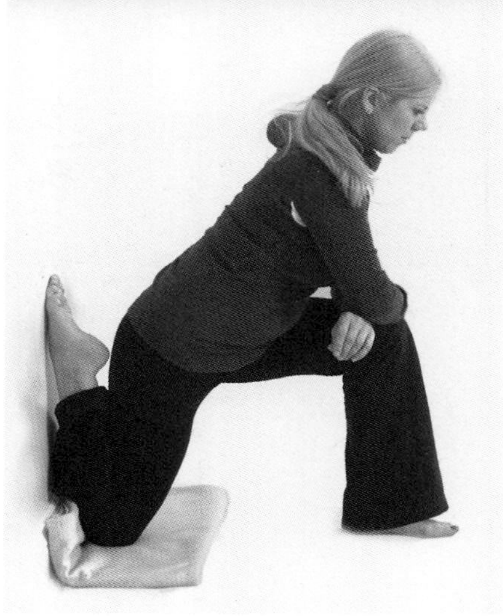
quad stretch series at the wall - 2

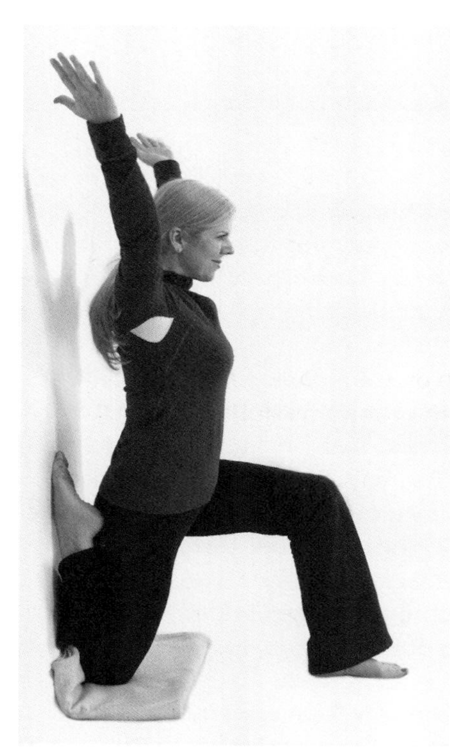
quad stretch series at the wall - 3

Ustrasana *or* Modified Ustrasana

Quad Stretch Series at the Wall

1. Place a folded blanket on floor against the wall.

2. Facing away from the wall, place the left knee at the base of the wall so that the front of the left lower leg is against the wall and the thigh faces away from it.

3. Supporting yourself with your hands, place the right foot flat on the floor so that you're in a shallow lunge. The right upper and lower leg form a 90 degree angle, with the right knee directly above the right ankle. The left knee and right foot should be hip width apart from left to right.

Before moving further, always ask why? Is it your ambition driving you, or is your body ready to let go?

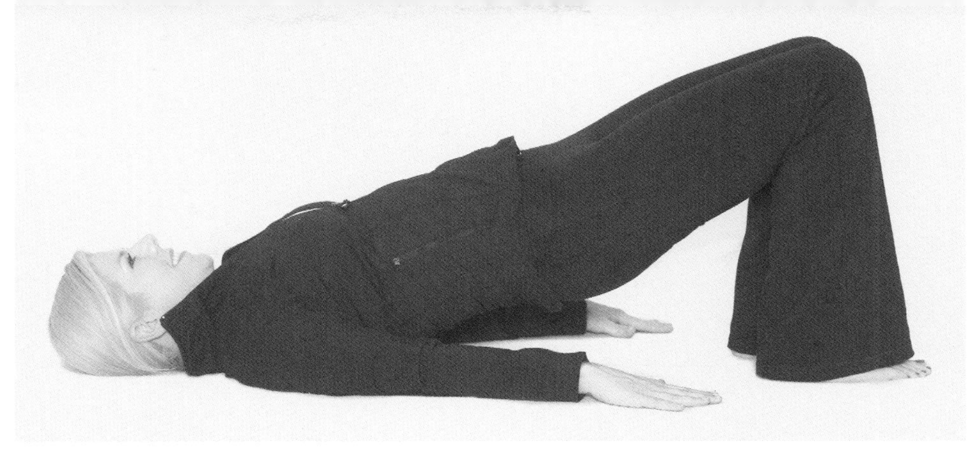

bridge pose

4. Supporting yourself on your hands, relax the shoulders and notice if there is a stretch in the left thigh. If more intensity is desired, slowly lift the torso to place the forearms on the right thigh. If more intensity is required, slowly take the arms overhead, palms facing each other and arm drawn into their shoulder sockets. There should be no sensations of spinal compression. Observe the sensations and breathe easy.

5. Return the hands to the floor if they aren't already there.

6. Slowly step the right foot forward a few inches and let the hips sink forward slightly into a lunge. If more intensity is desired explore the arm variations described above. Observe the sensations and breathe easy.

7. Come out of the pose, sit on the blanket with the legs extended forward and shake them out gently as you notice the sensations in both legs.

Change sides.

Ustrasana or *Modified Ustrasana*

Bridge Pose

1. Lie on the back with the knees bent and feet planted on the mat, hip width apart.

2. The knees are also hip width apart. The feet point straight forward and once the pelvis is lifted off the floor, the ankles are directly beneath the knees.

3. Lift the pelvis up on the exhale. Ensure that there is no sensation of compression, or stretch in the lower back. Stabilize, relax and breathe in the pose.

4. There should be equal pressure in the four corners of each foot.

5. Hold for ten easy breaths then gently release the pose.

Note:
The buttocks muscles will gently engage when you lift into Bridge Pose because the hips are moving into extension. Dicepher between tone and grip.

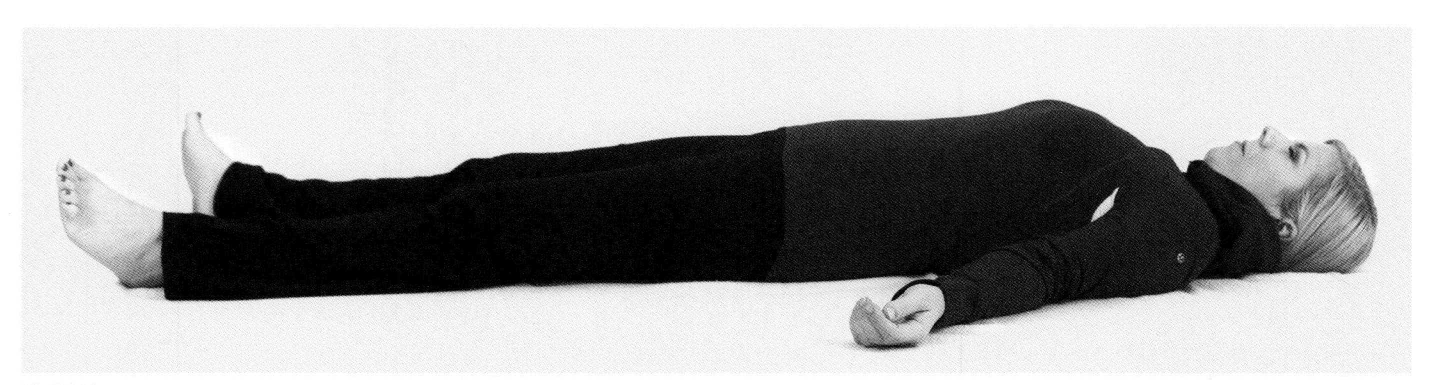

savasana

Ustrasana *or* Modified Ustrasana

Savasana

Breathe and feel the space within. Feel subtle energy flowing through your body. Soften into that energy, into the freedom within.

Questions to consider:
How did my body feel in the various positions? Which did it enjoy, and if so why? If not, why not? Did my stability, mobility and strength improve? Was I able to feel more? Am I able to differentiate between the feelings on opposites sides of my body? How does it feel to slow down and focus inward? What differences, subtle or obvious, can I feel in the pose from the first to the last instance? Do I think that I have a better awareness of the movement required to access this pose safely and effectively in my practice? Which exercise had the greatest impact, and why?

WE CAN MAKE OUR MINDS

SO LIKE STILL WATER

THAT BEINGS GATHER

ABOUT US,

THAT THEY MAY SEE

THEIR OWN IMAGES,

AND SO LIVE FOR A MOMENT

WITH A CLEARER,

PERHAPS EVEN WITH

A FIERCER LIFE

BECAUSE OF OUR QUIET.

—WILLIAM BUTLER YEATS

Advancing Your Practice

Here are some resources to help you continue to advance your practice.

ONLINE EDUCATION

Ask Susi: A Membership Based Site

"Ask Susi" is a resource for you to ask your questions about yoga, yoga and anatomy, yoga therapy, restorative yoga and finding language to cue effectively for your students. Here is some of what we have discussed — the ultimate hamstring releases; how to use the spinal strap; the best ways for moving into Uttanasana; working with sore outer ankles; how to release the thoracic spine; how to assess if a student is ready for shoulder stand; osteo-arthritic knees; how to work with someone in pain.

How it works: Send Susi your questions. Twice a month, Susi will host a teleclass to explore the questions asked. All calls are recorded so if you miss the call, you can tune in online. Calls are 1 hour in length. You will also have unlimited access to the exclusive Ask Susi website for the length of your subscription.

To register for "Ask Susi" email us at **iloveanatomy@anatomyandasana.com**.

Anatomy and Asana: Monthly Ezine to your Email Account

This is a free monthly ezine to further your understanding of Anatomy and Asana - a good burst of knowledge to incorporate into your practice, whether you are a teacher or student.

To receive this ezine, please visit **www.anatomyandasana.com**.

BOOKS, CDs, DVDs, STREAMING VIDEO

Susi has produced a number of books, cds, dvds and streaming video to support your practice whether you are a yoga student or yoga teacher. They focus on anatomy and therapeutic yoga and include the *Anatomy and Asana: Preventing Yoga Injury series; Therapeutic Yoga for the Shoulders and Hips, Yoga for the Desk Jockey*™, and *Finding Quiet*. To find out more, you can visit **www.functionalsynergy.com**.

LIVE WORKSHOPS

Susi has taught thousands of students and teachers concepts in anatomy and asana and therapeutic yoga. She offers a down-to-earth approach that is refreshing, fun, and easy to apply.

Workshops are offered as three hour mini-sessions; one day sessions, or three to five day trainings. For a full listing of trainings and workshops, please visit **www.anatomyandasana.com**.

Therapeutic Yoga for the Shoulders and Hips

Ever since Susi began teaching yoga, the two most common physical limitations she has seen are in the shoulders and hips. Even for people with back, neck, or knee pain, if they are able to improve the functioning of their shoulders and hips, their back or neck pain becomes much more manageable or even resolved.

In this workshop you will learn the biomechanics of the shoulders and hips, and how they impact each other; how they influence energy flow through the spine, and affect transfer of force and load from the upper body to the lower body and lower body to upper body. You'll learn therapeutic yoga asanas that improve the functioning of the shoulders and hips and improve the balance in and between your neck, mid back, and lower back. The result is less pain, less strain, and more freedom, stability and ease.

**Advancing Your Yoga Practice:
The Art of Slowing Down**

This workshop brings this book to life!

It is so easy to get lost and disconnected in yoga asanas, to become distracted by the "right way" to breathe and how to do each yoga asana properly. All of this tends to lead to more tightness, stiffness and over-gripping. In this workshop, you will experience the finesse of the asanas, making them work for your body, learning how each stimulus impacts and influences your sense of opening, release and stability. And, if you are a yoga teacher, you will learn ways to help your students stay connected, to help them let go of the "right way" and to feel the way their body wants to release and strengthen. It will enable you to answer the question, "How do I make the practice challenging enough to support and strengthen without over-extending?" The result – you will not only feel lighter and pain-free, you'll learn how to measure ease within your body.

For further details . . .

Call: **403-229-2617**
Email: **iloveanatomy@anatomyandasana.com**

Or visit our websites:
www.functionalsynergy.com
www.anatomyandasana.com

About Susi Hately Aldous

Susi Hately Aldous came to yoga as a result of her own injuries sustained from being a teenaged athlete. After four months of taking once weekly yoga classes, she was able to run a 10 K race pain-free. In the same time frame she was working as an exercise therapist at a multi-disciplinary rehabilitation clinic and began complementing her clients' programs with yoga. Her clients got better faster. With this experience she continued to study yoga and became certified in 1999.

In 1999, Susi established Functional Synergy and since 2001 has focused on customizing yoga programs for people with pain and injury and training teachers around the world in principles of anatomy and therapeutic yoga. Her diverse background, which includes a BSc. Kinesiology, yoga certification from India and Canada, training in mind-body medicine, and practical experience as an exercise therapist and ergonomics consultant, provides a functional and common sense approach to her teaching. Susi is also the author of *Anatomy and Asana: Preventing Yoga Injuries, Yoga for the Desk Jockey™*, and *Therapeutic Yoga for the Shoulders and Hips.*

TO CONTACT SUSI:

Phone: **403.229.2617**
Toll Free: **866.229.2645**
Email: **health@functionalsynergy.com**

About Leonor (Leo) Mowry

Originally, Leo started studying yoga as a means to combat stress in the corporate world. As she progressed in her practice, she realized many commonalities between yoga and her long-time study of Taoism. In 2001, Leo received her certification as an Interdisciplinary Yoga Teacher and left the corporate world to study and teach yoga, intent on extending her deepest personal beliefs to her professional life.

Leo owns and operates Village Yoga in Toronto, Canada. In addition to teaching group classes and private lessons, Leo specializes in teaching therapeutic yoga to students with various physical limitations and special needs. As her teaching journey progressed, Leo discovered a deep passion for therapeutic yoga and is continually gratified and amazed by the human capacity to heal, using simple techniques. She is the Yoga Director for the annual Toronto Trails Festival.

TO CONTACT LEONOR:

Phone: **416.487.2812**
Email: **info@villageyoga.ca**